D0003659

Twenty–One Days to
Health
THE HALLELUJAH DIET WAY

The nutritional and health information in this book is based on the teachings of God's Holy Word, the Bible, as well as research and personal experience by the author and others. The purpose of this book is to provide information and education about health. The author and publisher do not directly or indirectly dispense medical advice or prescribe the use of fasting or diet as a form of treatment for sickness without medical approval. Nutritionists and other experts in the field of health and nutrition hold widely varying views. The author and publisher do not intend to diagnose or prescribe. The author and publisher intend to offer health information to help you cooperate with your doctor or other health practitioner in your mutual quest for health. In the event you use this information without your doctor's or health practitioner's approval, you prescribe for yourself. This remains your constitutional right. The author and publisher assume no responsibility.

Contact Chet Day at chet@hacres.com
Visit our web site at http://www.hacres.com

First Printing 1998

ISBN 0-929619-08-0

This Edition Published and Distributed by:
Hallelujah Acres Publishing
PO Box 2388
Shelby, NC 28151
(704) 481-1700

Contents

Introduction

Welcome to a book that explains a diet and lifestyle program that may change your life more than you can possibly imagine in three short weeks.

Some men, women, and young adults (especially those with no apparent health problems) find our challenge to try the Hallelujah Diet for three months more than they can handle—after all, three months without meat, without sugar, without all the stuff we grow up thinking of as "good" sometimes seems like an eternity.

I mean, seriously, the thought of going a quarter of a year without a Snickers bar or a Dairy Queen soft serve or a plate of baby back ribs may indeed seem a bit much if you've never considered getting off the Standard American Diet before.

Well, to make the health changes you know you should make a little easier, Dr. George H. Malkmus—the founder of the Hallelujah Diet—and I invite you to try our *Twenty–One Day Contract to Health the Hallelujah Diet Way.*

That's right, three little ole weeks.

Now, three months sounds pretty tough, right?

But three weeks?

Hey, just about everybody can muster enough self–discipline to give up some favorite "foods" (which in actuality are killing you over the long term) for three weeks.

And if you're already on the Hallelujah Diet but have been cheating like a maniac because of the goodies well–meaning friends and relatives are always forcing down your throat every time you turn around, why not consider our *Twenty–One Day Contract to Health the Hallelujah Diet Way* and use it to do the diet 100% instead of only partially?

So, please, commit yourself to twenty–one days of fun and life–enhancement.

Okay, time for details on our *Twenty–One Day Contract to Health the Hallelujah Diet Way.*

To begin, I want to acknowledge my good friend and raw food brother, Dr. Robert Sniadach, who taught me the technique of the twenty–one day contract several years ago when I interviewed him for a newsletter I used to publish. Robert told me at the time:

• • •

"Let's talk about making twenty–one day commitments. Evidently some research suggests that twenty–one days is a good round figure for how long one needs to indulge in particular practices until they become sort of etched in our brains such that they suddenly become much easier for our whole body and system, physiology and neurology, to deal with, to accept as a more positive action. Almost like a habit, I guess. So I suggest that people make twenty–one day commitments for whatever goals they have in mind.

"Once you're able to practice a behavior for twenty–one days, it seems much easier to stick with. And twenty–one days isn't so long. Three weeks. Look at how many weeks you've been alive. Fifty–two weeks per year times however many years you've been alive, so when you just make a new commitment for three weeks it's not that big of a deal.

"Try your own little experiment and see how you do. This twenty–one day commitment seems to work pretty well for a lot of people. When my colleague Dr. Carol Cole and I work with people individually, we sit down and whip out a piece of pre–printed paper which we call a twenty–one–day contract, and we actually have our clients write down what it is they want to achieve and basically how they want to go about it, what steps they're going to take. We make sure it's an achievable goal without too much difficulty, and then we both sign it to the effect that it's now a contract in force that says that for the next twenty–one days our client will do such and such to reach a specific goal, and that we'll stay in contact every few days or so by phone or in person to make sure people are staying with their goal.

"Part of the deal is that they have to do this every day for twenty–one days. Susan Smith Jones talks about this a lot too, and she's had real good success with it. If people are able to stick with a behavior for those twenty–one days, many times it works out really well. If they don't stick with it for twenty–one days, if they slip up say on Day Nine, then they have to start over again and go for twenty–one consecutive days. That seems to be the key. So any slip up along the way means you have to start over—even if it's Day Twenty, you have to start over. Little patterns like this, little actions like this, help to build self–discipline and help to teach people just what they're capable of. And many times we pleasantly surprise ourselves with just what we are capable of doing."

• • •

Thank you, Dr. Sniadach.

Now, if what Robert just said makes sense to you, and it sure makes sense to me, won't you please photocopy the *Twenty–one Day Contract to Health the Hallelujah Diet Way* on page 6?

Sign it. Then get someone to witness it for you. By having a witness you eliminate at least a little of the wiggle room when temptations start rearing their ugly heads. Additionally, research into the lives of successful people has shown over and over again that writing down goals leads to success.

Wait, what's that? You say you don't want to sign a contract until you know just what you're getting into, that you want a quick review of the Hallelujah Diet?

Sure. Glad to oblige. See pages 98–99 for the complete Hallelujah Diet as taught by Dr. George H. Malkmus.

But, in a nutshell, for the next twenty–one days, to be on the Hallelujah Diet, you'll give up the five big killer foods we love so much in America: meat, dairy, sugar, white flour, and salt. You'll also give up coffee and all liquids other than freshly extracted juices and distilled water.

What do you mean, "Then what do I eat?"

Hey, for three wonderful weeks you're going to feed your body the foods that will revitalize it and make it hum like you wouldn't believe: you're going to feed it God's diet of predominently uncooked fruits and vegetables. You're also going to drink about sixteen ounces of fresh carrot/vegetable juice every day, and you'll have a few teaspoons or tablespoons of a "super green food" called Barleygreen. (If you need information about Barleygreen, turn to page 100.)

Oh yeah, we also recommend that you have one tablespoon a day of organic flax oil.

And for the evening meal you're going to have a big lettuce and vegetable salad followed by a delicious cooked supper consisting of things like whole grained pastas and breads, baked potatoes, yams, cornmeal muffins, brown rice, steamed vegetables, and so on.

Now that you know what you're getting into, let's turn our attention back to the paperwork.

Okay, here's your contract to health:

TWENTY–ONE DAY CONTRACT TO HEALTH THE HALLELUJAH DIET WAY

I, _____, do hereby contract with Hallelujah Acres to try the Hallelujah Diet for the next twenty–one days as taught by Dr. George Malkmus.

Below I list the goals or expectations I've set for myself during this period:

_____

_____

_____

_____

_____

_____

_____

Should I deviate from the terms of this contract during any one of the next twenty–one days, I will immediately start over again. I will adhere to the terms of this contract until I've completed a full twenty–one days on the Hallelujah Diet as specified above.

Signed _____

Witness _____

Date_____

Note: If you decide you have to qualify the diet (and this is appropriate and necessary in some circumstances), please don't qualify it with something like: "I will have three scoops of Breyer's Chocolate Mint ice cream at nine p.m. every day." An appropriate qualification would be something like, "Since I have severe candida I will not eat fruit" or "Since I am an insulin–dependent diabetic I will not have much fruit or carrot juice and will carefully monitor my blood sugar several times a day."

The purpose of the program is to go as close to 100% on the diet as you reasonably can at this time, given your general health conditions. And of course we recommend that you go on our program with the help and guidance of your nutritionally aware physician or health counselor or local health minister who has trained at Hallelujah Acres.

When do you start your contract?

As soon as possible.

This gives you plenty of time to get to the store or farmer's market to stock up on fresh fruits and vegetables and to track down a juicer to borrow if you don't already have one. I assume you already have a jar of Barleygreen. If you don't, you can order one now and start using it as soon as it arrives. (See page 100.)

Or if you don't have the money or have some kind of objection to using a health product, you can write in as your qualifier that you'll follow a fruit/vegetable/juice diet but without Barleygreen. (Though we certainly urge you not to do that since we consider Barleygreen one of the three dietary keys to the success of our health program.)

To help you succeed with our *Twenty–One Day Contract to Health the Hallelujah Diet Way*, I've provided in this book a daily motivational "how to" letter. There are twenty–one days of these letters and each letter provides many details which explain how to properly practice the Hallelujah Diet and lifestyle.

For example, in these daily letters I cover what to expect when you start, how to juice, how to prepare salads, how to develop an exercise program, how to get some sunshine each day, how to stay motivated, how to make excellent use of prayer and meditation time, and so on.

Whoa, it'll be like getting daily individual coaching every 24 hours for three weeks.

(As another motivational factor, let me add that you could easily spend several hundred dollars, probably even a grand, to get the kind of coaching and nutritional/lifestyle information from some doctor, weight loss clinic, health coach, or nutritional expert that you'll read in the remaining pages of this book.)

Come on, my friend, with the knowledge in this book you have a chance to start building a new you for the next century, and you may be only twenty–one days away from feeling the best you've ever felt.

So xerox that contract, fill it in, sign it and have someone witness it, and let's have some fun as we build a new you.

Since you'll drink an ocean of juices during your *Twenty–One Day Contract to Health the Hallelujah Diet Way*, I want to share my favorite juice recipe with you.

• • •

Chet's Carrot Concoction

I recently retired my Champion and purchased a Green Power Juicer and have been giving it a great workout. Just about every day of my life, I prepare the following favorite drink:

5 huge juicing carrots
3 stalks of celery (cut in 1" pieces)
2–3 leaves of Romaine lettuce
1 medium Granny Smith or Fuji apple

Peel the carrots and the apple. Run all through your Green Power or Champion juicer. Makes a bit more than 16–ounces. Have eight ounces immediately and store the rest in a tightly sealed jar to drink later. As Dr. Malkmus says in his seminar, your cells will be shouting "Whooooeeeeee" as they assimilate this flood of good nutrients.

• • •

Okay, enough with the introduction. Go buy the supplies you need and stock that frig of yours with the best produce you can find and get ready to change your life.

Note: You'll have more fun with your Twenty–one Day Contract if you read each day's letter on the appropriate day. Don't read ahead.

Day One of Our Twenty–One Days to Health the Hallelujah Diet Way

Good morning, and thank you for joining me on this exciting 21–day adventure to better health.

I hope you're as enthusiastic and excited about this journey as I am, and I want to personally thank you for making this choice for life and for health.

By committing to this contract, you are part of a grassroots movement that has the potential to literally eliminate sickness in America and around the world. Hallelujah!

Regarding mechanics of the contract, each morning for the next three weeks, you should read that particular day's letter of encouragement. Each letter will provide motivation and support that'll help you achieve the goals you set forth in your contract.

For our first day, I want to encourage you to maintain your spirit of fun while also recognizing that your body will go through some exciting changes during the next twenty–one days and especially during the first week.

If you adhere closely to the diet, your body will begin to cleanse itself and unload some of the toxins it's been carrying around in the bloodstream and in various pockets in muscles, tissues, and organs. During this detox period, you may experience a variety of symptoms, everything from headache to weakness. It's normal to experience symptoms, so don't draw the conclusion, "Oh mercy, this diet's making me sick."

No, my friend, eating fruits and vegetables, and drinking carrot juice and Barleygreen, and getting some gentle exercise won't make you sick. But doing so *will* provide your body with the nutrients it needs to start cleansing itself of the junk that has accumulated from years of less than perfect living.

If you want more details on symptoms, please read Chapter Nine, "The Healing Crisis," in *Recipes for Life…from God's Garden* or Chapter 23 in *God's Way to Ultimate Health* (see page 100 for info on how to order these books).

These transitory symptoms represent the major downside of upgrading your diet. Many people just won't feel so hot the first few days of diet changes. And a few won't feel so hot for the first week or even longer. But, happily, these symptoms do pass pretty rapidly in most cases. And some won't experience any cleansing symptoms at all.

When people have more symptoms than they want to have, we encourage them to slow down the detox process by having less Barleygreen and less carrot juice and by eating more cooked food at the evening meal. Taking any or all three of these actions will slow down the body's release of stored toxins.

The big advantage of going through the detox process is incredible because most people just plain feel better and better once the body starts cleansing and renewing itself.

Please remember that it takes months and years of poor living to get in mediocre health, and you can't regain ideal health overnight. Yes, the body heals itself, but obviously it can't totally rebuild itself in a few days.

So, *be patient* with yourself and recognize that you may not feel so great during the initial days of this experience.

If you do have some symptoms, be thankful because symptoms mean your body's getting rid of stuff that it doesn't want inside it. Better outside the body than in, eh?

Okay, enough about symptoms.

When they first get on the Hallelujah Diet, many people want some kind of outline to follow as to what to eat and what to do during the day.

To give you some idea of a sample program, here's my health and menu plan for Day One of the twenty–one day contract:

Every day of my life between 4:30 and 6 a.m., I wake up fully and naturally without an alarm clock. Practically humming with energy and enthusiasm, I can't wait to get at the day's activities. Before I stopped getting sick by changing my diet and lifestyle, I ate a huge breakfast. Not any more. Here's how I eat now:

Breakfast
Tablespoon of Barleygreen (beginners should start with a teaspoon). I take my Barleygreen straight from the bottle, but most will prefer to have it mixed in a couple ounces of distilled water.

Mid–morning
8 ounces of freshly extracted juice composed of two or three very large carrots (try to purchase California–grown "Bunny Luv" carrots if you can find them) and a Granny Smith apple (Dr. Malkmus prefers his carrot juice without the apple).

Lunch
Tablespoon of Barleygreen (beginners should start with a teaspoon), followed 20–30 minutes later by a couple of navel oranges.

Mid–afternoon
If hungry, I'll snack on a handful or two of organic raisins.

Late afternoon
Slow jogging (11–12 minute miles) or rebounding for 20–30 minutes followed by 20 minutes of weight lifting with light weights.

Early evening
When I finish exercising, I'll immediately have a tablespoon of Barleygreen (beginners should start with a teaspoon) before I get in the shower. After shower-ing, I'll make another 8–10 ounces of freshly extracted juice (a couple of very

large carrots, Granny Smith apple, a stalk or two of celery, and a Romaine lettuce leaf or two). Yummy.

Supper

Large blended salad (four Romaine lettuce leaves, one medium tomato, one half Haas avocado, three stalks of celery, one medium carrot—put tomato and avocado in blender and blend—then add lettuce and carrots, pushing down with celery stalk—blend until smooth and then eat like a cold soup).

While the salad is digesting, I'll make a simple supper of brown rice and steamed vegetables (cauliflower, broccoli, green beans, carrots, whatever I have in the vegetable bin that looks good to me).

I end the day by meditating for 30 minutes (I'll provide details on how you can use prayer/meditation as part of your health routine in the Day Twelve letter). I'm in bed by 10:30 or 11 p.m. and sound asleep in a matter of minutes.

And that will be it for my routine for today.

Although you can try my program, you should immediately start working on developing your own. We have some great recipes on our web site at *http://www.hacres.com* so please make use of them.

Also, do remember that we're all different, and each of us will require more or less food.

You should not be hungry on the Hallelujah Diet.

Eat all you want—it's just about impossible to overeat on fruits and vegetables. And most people will be amazed at how little hunger they experience on this diet.

You know why? Because the body's finally getting the nutrition it needs instead of the almost total lack of nutrition found in the Standard American Diet of dead "foods."

Note, however, that it's easy to overeat on fruits, so we do recommend that you monitor yourself and not go overboard by eating 10–20 pieces of fruit every 24 hours. I rarely have more than 4–5 pieces of fruit in any given day, and I feel a lot better than a few years ago when I ate way too much of the wonderful stuff. These days I concentrate on putting the vegetable "healthy cell builders" in my body.

Also note that exercise is a fundamental part of the Hallelujah Diet and lifestyle. I'll have some tips on exercise programs in tomorrow's letter.

Until then, thank you again for joining me with the *Twenty–One Day Contract to Health the Hallelujah Diet Way.*

I hope you're having as much fun on this adventure as I am.

See you tomorrow.

Day Two of Our Twenty–One Days to Health the Hallelujah Diet Way

Good morning.

Welcome to Day Two, and I hope you feel great about getting past the big hump of the first day of your contract.

In my experience with various detoxing programs the past several years, the initial three to four days are the hardest because the body goes through intense changes as it switches over from the Standard American Diet (SAD) of processed "foods" to natural foods that the body can efficiently utilize for health and rejuvenation. When we're drinking carrot juice, eating predominently uncooked fruits and vegetables, and having some Barleygreen, our trillions of cells, as Dr. Malkmus says, begin yelling: "Whoooeee! At last you've given me something to build some new healthy, vital, vibrant cells with!" And as the new strong cells start building, the body has to flush out the old, weak cells, along with various pockets of toxic material that it's been storing.

The result of this process?

The various symptoms we talked about yesterday. I got a wonderful letter in the mail the second morning when I did this contract challenge on the Internet. A lady wrote, *"I want to thank you for your encouragement regarding the detox process. I started the Hallelujah Diet right after I finished the books my mom–in–law gave me for Christmas, and I said to my husband the other day that I felt like I had been POISONED (and I haven't even gotten any Barleygreen yet). That's the only way to describe the horrible nausea, weakness, and general malaise. It's starting to pass now—thankfully, and my prayer continues to be that I can do all things through Christ who gives me strength."*

I share this letter with you because it expresses so well what some people experience with the first few days of going on the Hallelujah Diet—what the alternative health movement calls a "healing crisis." Happily, once these initial poisons leave the body, most people start to feel better and better. The secret is to either ride out the hours or days of weakness, malaise, nausea, rashes, and so on or else to slow down the elimination process by cutting back on the Barleygreen, cutting back on the amount of juice, and/or adding more cooked food at the evening meal.

Okay, enough about that. Just wanted to reiterate the point since I know you may be having second thoughts about now because you're feeling worse than you felt when you started the program.

Please remember, you have to pass through winter to get to spring.

Now to today's topic: exercise.

I've been working like a maniac at Hallelujah Acres the past couple of weeks and yesterday I was very involved with this 21–day project as well as with another major project as well as with a huge influx of e–mail, and, during the day as the hours flew past, I kept thinking, "How am I going to have time to exercise this afternoon?"

Well, four p.m. rolled around, and I still hadn't finished the projects I wanted to finish, but I thought about my personal 21–day contract, and I thought about how I wouldn't want to confess in today's letter that I didn't do my exercise, so I dropped everything and went home and jogged for twenty minutes and then lifted weights for twenty minutes, and, you know what?

The decision to stop working and go exercise was the best decision I'd made in over a month.

You see, it's also a decision I hadn't been making often enough lately because I've just been too busy to get out and exercise every day.

Well, not anymore.

I felt so good after that exercise yesterday that I rededicated myself to getting in my daily jog or weightlifting or rebounding or whatever no matter how busy I was or how many interesting projects pulled at me.

Why is it so important to exercise, you ask?

Well, remember that when you change your diet, your body starts to excrete toxins and poisons that it's stored in various places throughout the system.

Exercise helps to remove this gunk.

Think about sweating for a moment. When you sweat, your body has about a zillion pores that it can use to push garbage out of your system. So doesn't it make sense to work up a sweat and give the body this excellent avenue for moving the junk out?

And that's not to mention the fact that exercising gets highly oxygenated blood moving throughout the system, bringing life–giving oxygen to areas that may have been oxygen–deprived for years because of sedentary habits.

I've found with my personal program that exercise is just about as important to good health as diet.

So what do you do if you haven't exercised since high school?

Do you go out on the local track and run a fast mile? Do you challenge Michael Jordan to a game of pick–up? Do you ask Mike Tyson to spar a few rounds with you?

Of course not. Doing one of those things if you're not in shape would either put you down on exercise forever or it might even kill you.

Please approach exercise the same way you approach the Hallelujah Diet. We teach that with exercise you do the same thing as with the diet—you make a commitment to your health and to your body/temple and then you follow through.

Dr. Malkmus teaches in his seminars that the best way to start a daily exercise program is to go outside and measure off one mile. Then walk that mile as briskly as you can (if an entire mile is too much for you, and you get tired or sore, walk as much as you can comfortably and then stop). Time how long it takes you to do this mile or whatever distance you can cover comfortably.

Now shout *Hallelujah* because you've just completed your exercise for the day.

The next day, go outside and do the same mile but try to cover its distance in a shorter time. When you can do that mile in fifteen minutes, you add a second mile. Your eventual goal is to cover four miles in less than an hour, and if you do this at least five times a week, you're going to give your body one more edge in its God-given tendency of seeking health.

And if you're into jogging, go for it. Or rebounding. Or swimming. Or bicycling. Studies prove that folks who get at least 20 minutes of aerobic exercise every day live longer than folks who don't. So make exercise a required part of your daily health program.

If you can't find the time, do what I did yesterday: put the work off and *make* the time for you today. The work will still be there tomorrow, I promise.

And we don't have the same assurance about ourselves, do we? So make time for your health—it's the most important time you'll spend every day of your life.

Regarding other types of exercise, Dr. Malkmus and I both recommend some resistance or weight training as being very healthy for people. We don't mean to start doing squats with 400 lbs. of iron—that would be like sparring with Mike Tyson again—you wouldn't last very long.

We're talking about a gentle, slowly progressing program of toning and strengthening the body's muscles. I use a cheapo set of weights that I purchased at Wal-Mart for under $30. As for what to do with the weights, I'll leave that up to you. There are a quadrillion different ways of pumping iron, and each of us needs to pick out the routines that make us feel the best. Check the local library, bookstore, or Internet for details.

When I'm not being a workaholic and am in decent shape, my exercise routine goes like this: I lift three days a week with a 20-minute jog afterwards. On days when I don't lift, I jog or rebound for about an hour. I take Sundays off. Every day, I warm-up with a few minutes of stretching and rebounding.

If you don't have 30–60 minutes a day set aside for some kind of exercise (even if it's just walking in the fresh air), then you need to start doing it right now.

Chet's health plan for Day Two:

Breakfast
Tablespoon of Barleygreen (beginners should start with a teaspoon). I take my Barleygreen straight from the bottle, but most will prefer to have it mixed in a couple ounces of distilled water.

Mid-morning
8 ounces of freshly extracted juice (two very large carrots and a Granny Smith apple)

Lunch
Tablespoon of Barleygreen (beginners should start with a teaspoon), followed 20 minutes later by several bananas.

Mid–afternoon
If hungry, I'll snack on a handful or two of organic raisins or a couple of slices of dried pineapple or a handful of dehydrated apricots.

Late afternoon
Slow jogging (11–12 minute miles) for 30 to 45 minutes.

Early evening
When I finish exercising, I'll immediately have a tablespoon of Barleygreen (beginners should start with a teaspoon) before I get in the shower. After showering, I'll make another 8–10 ounces of freshly extracted juice (a couple of very large carrots, Granny Smith apple, a stalk of celery, and a Romaine lettuce leaf or two). Yummy.

Supper
Large blended salad (four Romaine lettuce leaves, one medium tomato, one half Haas avocado, three stalks of celery, one medium carrot—put tomato and avocado in blender and blend—then add lettuce and carrots, pushing down with celery stalk—blend until smooth and then eat like a cold soup).

While the salad is digesting, I'll make a simple supper of a large baked Idaho potato stuffed with three–day old sunflower and red and green lentil sprouts. I'll top this weird–sounding but delicious tasting concoction with a sprinkle of dulse (a dried sea vegetable like kelp which is available at most health food stores). If this combination sounds good to you, make a note on your shopping list to pick up some organic lentils and sunflower seeds. You have plenty of time during the next twenty–one days to do a little sprouting.

(If you don't know how to do this, put two heaping tablespoons of sunflower seeds and two heaping tablespoons of lentils in a canning jar. Cover with a couple inches of distilled water. After four hours, pour off the water. In the evening, rinse the seeds with water, swirling it around vigorously, and then pour off the water. Do the same thing the next morning. Do the same thing the next evening. Repeat this process until the tails of the sprouts are at least as long as the seeds themselves. Then do one final rinse, pour off the water, and refrigerate. Sprouts keep a few days, but they're the most enzymatically active just before you put them in the icebox.)

I'll end the day by meditating for 30 minutes.

That takes care of Day Two.

Tomorrow I want to write more about how the body eliminates toxins and what you can do to speed up the process.

If you're having some symptoms here on Day Two, remember that you're not alone.

With tens of thousands of copies of *Twenty–One Days to Health the Hallelujah Diet Way* in either print or Internet file format, you can rest assured that you're in good company.

My friend, we all sit together in the same boat, and isn't it wonderful that so many have made a commitment to improving their health?

Seriously, it gives me and Dr. Malkmus goosebumps when we talk about how blessed we are to have the chance to share what we've learned about health with so many others who will then go out and share what they've learned.

We can make a difference. We can heal this sick and suffering world. Whoa, isn't it hugely exciting?

Enough excitement. It's too early for me to get this pumped up. Actually, when you practice the Hallelujah Diet and lifestyle program, you end up being this pumped up and energetic ALL the time.

Man, it's something else, believe me.

Anyway, please hang in there and stick with your contract even if you're not feeling so hot today because if you're like most people you're going to feel a whole LOT better in a day or two or three, and then you'll be so glad you didn't stop the perfectly natural process of healing that your body's undergoing.

See you tomorrow, Day Three of our *Twenty–One Day Contract to Health the Hallelujah Diet Way*.

Day Three of Our Twenty–One Days to Health the Hallelujah Diet Way

Good morning.

Welcome to Day Three, and I hope you're feeling better today than you felt yesterday.

Before I get started on today's topic—elimination—I want to address those who may have "slipped" in meeting the terms of your contract.

First, and most important, do not beat up on yourself.

Dietary and lifestyle changes do not come easily. Habits of a lifetime don't disappear overnight.

Please recognize that every individual who starts the health journey takes forward steps and backward steps. I've been walking this path for five years, and I still stumble on occasion—though I don't fall very often anymore.

When I make a choice I later regret, I smile and gently remind myself to try to do better with the next choice. Then I let go of the poor choice and move on.

We only live in the moment, my friend, and we can't do much about past moments other than to learn from them, so there's no reason to dwell on mistakes or to be mean to yourself about choices you regret.

Instead of letting those past moments affect you, why not love yourself and recognize your humanity instead?

Remember, God loves you, your family loves you, and friends love you, warts and all.

So respond to yourself with love and move on happily and with a desire to do better the next time.

Okay, a few words about elimination.

If you are of delicate sensibilities, you may want to skim past the next few pages since I'm going to discuss bowel movements and urination.

Yuck.

I don't bring up this subject when formally dining with someone like Amy Vanderbilt, but because of the importance of the topic I need to mention it at this point in our twenty–one day journey to health.

To get into the flow of this, let's start with urine. As major organs of elimination, your kidneys will work overtime during this twenty–one day period as they filter all kinds of heavy metals and toxic materials out of the bloodstream. Consequently, you need to drink plenty of water and juices to keep things moving. People like Dr. Weil and the other media docs tell you to drink at least eight 8–oz. glasses of water every day.

Good idea, though we'd qualify it by saying you should have a combination of distilled water and freshly extracted juices. Shoot for consuming about 64–oz. total each day. Personally, I try to consume 16–oz. of carrot juice and the rest distilled water every day of my life.

Okay, let's move from urine to—well, let's move on—err, next topic, please.

You see, when some people change their diet, they also experience constipation. Although not unusual, no one finds constipation pleasant.

First off, recognize that most Americans, indeed most people in the world not living natural lives, suffer almost constant constipation.

Whoa, say what?

Well, if you don't have at least two copious and fast bowel movements every day, unless you have a very unusual system, you're one of the millions on this planet who suffers from chronic constipation.

Did you know that everything you eat, from the moment it enters your mouth until the moment it leaves your body, should be processed and cleared from your system in less than 24 hours?

Did you know that meat can take up to 48 hours to go through the body?

Think about leaving a hamburger patty in your crock pot at the temperature of 98.6 degrees for 48 hours.

Lift off the lid and take a whiff.

Peeeeuuuuuu!

Now you know why most people leave odiferous calling cards in restrooms. Now you know why most people have body odor and bad breath.

Wonder about your personal bowel transit time? Here's an easy way to find out: when you make your next salad, grate a beet in with it. Keep an eye on your stool—no, not your footstool—but the stuff…never mind.

Anyway, when you see a reddish stool, you'll know your bowel transit time. Ideally it should be between 12 and 24 hours.

Most people aren't anywhere near that.

Without being gross, when you're not constipated, you sit down on the commode, you unload your baggage in a matter of seconds, and you're up and about your business. No straining, no waiting, no fuss, no muss. Just a tremendously satisfying "whoosh," and you're flushing before you know it.

I kid you not.

You'll be amazed at both the size and speed of your daily elimination. (Oh man, there go those happy hours of reading on the john.)

But most people have never had an unconstipated bowel movement and wouldn't recognize one if it hit them on the head.

Err, let's rephrase that…and wouldn't recognize one if they had one.

Anyway, you can do some things to help speed up your elimination of toxins, both through your kidneys and your large intestines, and here are a few options for your information and consideration:

1. Drink plenty of juice and distilled water. The more pure water you drink during your early days of diet and lifestyle changes, the better. Having plenty of water in your system will not only help constipation, but it will also help the kidneys do their job and filter gunk out of the bloodstream.

2. Eat buckets of salad with lots and lots of leafy green lettuces and veggies (Romaine, bok choy, cabbage, leaf lettuce, and so on). The fiber in salad veggies works very efficiently as "nature's broom" to help clean the organs of digestion and elimination.

2. Be wary of eating too much fruit because fruit can constipate. I didn't realize this when I first started my diet changes, and it took me a long time to understand that even though I was practically living on fruit I needed the cellulose in vegetables to have healthy bowel movements. If you're from Missouri and like to see for yourself, go two days on fruit alone and then go two days on blended salads (or regular) salads. If you don't see the difference, I'll eat my hat. (Well, not really. Hats aren't on the Hallelujah Diet.)

4. Supplement your diet with a natural product like Herbal Fiberblend or psyllium powder to add even more bulk to your system. Don't overdo with these products, however, as they can cause bloating and gas in some folks, especially when first using them. We recommend the use of Herbal Fiberblend, and most of us at Hallelujah Acres use it daily. (See page 100 for details on Herbal Fiberblend.)

Okay, okay, enough about elimination. Put an end to it, Chet!

Let's turn now to three good letters that came in when I did this contract challenge in early 1998 on the Internet:

• • •

Dear Chet:

If I believed in doctors, I'd say you were just what the doctor ordered.

It was Day Two, 4 p.m. I was feeling crappy and in the process of giving up, deciding not to go to my ice–skating lesson at 5:30 p.m., not to spend time on organizing another salad, etc.

Then I remembered to check for your message. And you saved me.

One, you reminded me that "crappy" was good (healing crisis) and two, you recounted your four o'clock exercise story. That's when I remembered that I hadn't exercised yet.

So I did (skating lesson), and I felt great later.

Chet, I have to say it: When you're right, you're right. And right on target, too!

• • •

Chet, I just had to write and tell you that your encouragement e–mail came at a critical time for me. I had so many aches and pains, as well as a sinus headache, I thought I had the flu, and I prayed for the Lord's direction as to whether I should continue on the diet. When I read your first letter and realized the cause, I had to Praise the Lord for the timing of it. The mailman brought me a confirmation of my order for Barleygreen and the testimony of a man who had been healed of cancer. He wrote that he had had surgery for prostate cancer and was told that he would have to have his bladder removed as well. He went on the juice and Barleygreen diet instead, and one year later, his doctors told him he had no cancer at all. Praise the Lord again. That afternoon, my husband sat with me and watched a video of Dr. Malkmus' seminar and was so enthusiastic, he said he wanted to start on the diet as well. Talk about an answer to prayer! Needless to say, I am very encouraged, and feeling better.

• • •

Hey, Chet—you might make a bigger plug for rebounding. Even if people only do VERY mild rebounding to start, it is very helpful re: lymphatic movement. Each time you are at the top of your bounce, you are temporarily weightless and most all muscles are relaxed. Then at the bottom of your bounce, you are at 2 to 3 G's, plus most all your muscles must contract in order to rebalance yourself on the flexible surface of the rebounder as you make contact. So all this equals a tremendous, body–wide muscle contraction that pumps the dickens out of lymphatic fluid. Even light bouncing helps a lot.—Dr. Robert Sniadach

• • •

Regarding my personal health program for Day Three, other than a different lunch and dinner, it'll be identical to the past two days, so I won't repeat it here. Besides, by this point you should be getting comfortable making your own food choices from the Hallelujah Diet (see pages 98–99 for details).

Just think, you're almost halfway through the first week already. Golly, time sure flies when you're having fun, doesn't it?

See you tomorrow.

Day Four of Our Twenty–One Days to Health the Hallelujah Diet Way

Good morning.

Welcome to Day Four, and I hope you're feeling better today than you felt yesterday. Just think, by the time you read this we'll be halfway through our first week, and you've probably already had a pound or two of excess lard melt away from your body .

As I write these words, it's a little after six on a Thursday morning, and it's raining felines and canines here in Shelby, North Carolina. Muggy and hot, I feel like I'm back in Florida. I'll be glad when the weather turns cold again, and we get back to winter.

Mercy, El Niño has sure played havoc with the weather, hasn't it?

But I'll spare you my opinions regarding the El Niño phenomenon.

Let's get down to some serious Hallelujah Health Building, shall we?

Today I want to say a few more words in favor of blended salads.

Both of my major health mentors, Dr. George Malkmus and Dr. Stanley S. Bass, enjoy blended salads and recommend them as being an excellent addition to the human diet.

Why?

Because a blended salad has its ingredients processed into almost a liquid, and consequently you'll absorb more of the nutrients. Remember that if you don't chew thoroughly—and most Americans gulp their meals rather than chewing them—you're not eating properly.

The blended salad overcomes masticating mishaps because a machine does the chewing for you.

Remember also, however, that you still need to swirl the salad around your tongue and between your teeth to allow it to mix with saliva for at least some mouth digestion too.

Do you look and sound like a cow when you eat blended salad properly?

Well, you sure can if you're dining alone—and I slurp and slobber and swirl like the best cow in a green pasture when my wife and kids aren't with me—but you can also eat a blended salad quite delicately if you mind your manners. Just pretend you're supping with Amy Vanderbilt.

Moooo!

How do you make a blended salad?

Simple.

Let me walk you through my basic recipe: in my cheapo Waring blender, I drop in a tomato which I have either quartered or whacked into eighths, depending on the size. On top of the tomato pieces, I drop in one small, quartered baby cucumber (usually about the size of two thumbs in length). I hit the grind button and turn these two ingredients into mush. Let me add that I peel the waxed part off the cucumber. (In fact, with the exception of bell peppers, I run the peeler over everything that has a hint of wax on it since I don't want that junk gunking up my insides.)

Now it's time for a teaspoon of dulse (a sea vegetable like kelp that you can purchase in a flaked form at your local health food store). Then I add half of a bell pepper (green or red). Next come four to eight leaves of Romaine or other green–leaf lettuce. At this time, I also toss in anything else in the vegetable bin that looks good to me—some broccoli or cauliflower florets, a little turnip, a handful of snow peas, half an avocado—you decide.

Pack all this stuff loosely into the blender. Now pull off three or four good–sized celery stalks to add one at a time. (Don't forget to wash your produce.)

Turn the blender on to *grind* or *chop* or whatever speed works for you, and use the celery stalks to gently push the other ingredients into the blades. After some mild exclamations of frustration (no cursing, of course), the whole deal will eventually wind up as a liquefied mass that doesn't look very appetizing.

Don't worry—the first blended salad is the hardest to make. After you get the hang of it, you can make one of these in a matter of minutes, and if your family's not around or you're not dining at the Vanderbilts, you can even stand right at the kitchen counter and drink your salad out of the blender container.

Of course the more delicate and socially mature will not choose this option.

(Lest you fear I am not delicate and socially mature, I want to put that misconception to rest here and now. My friends, I know how to use two forks at a meal and don't think they were put there so I could use one with each hand at the same time. But, as you've probably guessed by now, Type–A that I am, I also like to save precious minutes, and sipping salad out of the blender does save a few minutes. And if nobody else is around, what's the harm, eh?)

Regarding appearance of your blended salad, during my early days with the concoctions, my wife and kids ran around the kitchen yelling, "Yuck, you're going to eat THAT?" These days they aren't so vocal, and I can even get them to try a bite or two once in a while.

But, for the most part, when they make fun of my blended salad, I just give them my most superior smile and nod sagely.

Little do they know what they're missing, both in terms of taste and nutrition.

So don't throw your blended salad away just because it looks like baby poop and because your family makes fun of you.

Instead, pour it into your finest crystal bowl, pull out one of your best spoons from the silver cabinet, and then sit in a quiet environment and enjoy a remarkably healthy and flavorful treat. Not only will you enjoy the taste (experiment with ingredients until you find combinations that make your taste buds yell "Wow!"), but you'll also assimilate more vitamins, minerals, and other nutrients than you would have had you chewed the ingredients separately.

I should add that tossing in a peeled apple also makes a wonderful addition, especially for those with a sweet tooth.

Oh yeah, if you can find a decent, ripe avocado, peel that baby and then toss it in too.

Whoa, you've never had anything taste this good.

Well, that 16–oz. filet mignon grilled in clarified butter and topped with fresh lemon pepper and followed by a huge piece of New York cherry cheese cake that you used to eat in the old days might come close.

Just kidding—and if the thought of eating a steak and a piece of cheese cake now makes you a little squeamish, you know you're on the right track with the Hallelujah Diet.

Okay, with today's letter I want to share a recipe. Let's begin with Rhonda Malkmus' delicious and all–raw…

• • •

Sunflower Loaf

1 cup hulled sunflower seeds
1 cup almonds
1 cup pumpkin seeds
1/2 red pepper
1/4 cup parsley
1/2 red onion
1 garlic clove
1 carrot

Soak seeds and almonds overnight and drain. In food processor with an S blade, a Green Power using the blank and with the least amount of tension, or a Champion Juicer with the blank in place, put the seeds, carrot, garlic, and almonds through. To this mixture, add the minced parsley, finely chopped red pepper, and onion.

Make a sauce of the following in a blender or food processor:

2 medium tomatoes
2 Tbsp. Bragg Liquid Aminos (optional)
1 Tbsp. basil
1 Tbsp. oregano

Mix half of the sauce into the loaf mixture, form into loaf and cover and set aside unrefrigerated for 4 to 6 hours. (The longer this loaf is allowed to marinate, the stronger the flavors become.) To serve, place the loaf on a bed of lettuce and pour the remaining tomato mixture over the top.

• • •

Okay, that's about it for Day Four. I trust you're doing well and starting to feel more energetic. If not, continue to be patient and remind yourself that the body can't heal itself in 3.5 days when you've probably spent a life time nourishing it on processed and junk foods that just plain don't sustain health.

And if you didn't find time for at least 10–20 minutes of some kind of exercise yesterday, please do so today.

See you tomorrow.

Day Five of Our Twenty–One Day Contract to Health the Hallelujah Diet Way

Good morning, fellow Hallelujah Health Seekers.

I popped out of bed at 4:30 this morning, bursting with energy and eager to get to my mail. You can't imagine how gratifying it is to open an e–mail box every morning to find it stuffed with great letters like this one:

• • •

My mother, Mary, was told last Christmas that she had terminal cancer. The doctors sent her home to die. She got on Dr. Malkmus's diet and I am proud to say she is well on her way to being cancer free. I am drinking my carrot juice as I am sending this note. Thanks for everything. The web site is great.

• • •

Today, feeling even more feisty than usual, I want to rather vocally address the issue of the liquids we put in our bodies.

I can state the Hallelujah Acres' position on this topic very clearly: Drink nothing but freshly extracted fruit and vegetable juices and distilled water.

As Dr. Norman Walker taught many years ago, the best liquid we can put in our bodies, bar none, comes from freshly extracted juices. Nature has distilled this water and added to it the nutrients needed to not only sustain life but also to activate our God–given immune systems. As Dr. Malkmus says in his seminars, these liquids make our cells shout, "Whoooeeee!"

Just as an automobile performs best on a good grade of gasoline, our bodies hum and purr when we fuel them with predominently uncooked fruits and vegetables and the juices extracted from them.

You want the engine in your car to knock and ping and lose efficiency and eventually clog up?

Then put cheap gas from some no–name convenience store in the tank every week.

The same holds true for your body.

If you want to clog up your arteries, fuel them on dead animal flesh and milk, which Dr. Malkmus so aptly calls "liquid meat." Add some sugar and white flour every meal and rattle the salt shaker over everything except the chocolate cake for dessert, and you have the recipe for chronic health problems as you age.

So here at Hallelujah Acres we teach people to only put life–enhancing liquids in their bodies.

Why do we condemn soft drinks and coffee?

That's a legitimate question since most Americans just plain can't get started in the morning without their coffee. And most of them can't get through the day without a can or three of Coke or Tab or Pepsi or Dr. Pepper or Surge or Jolt.

Hey, I speak with authority on today's topic because for years and years I fueled my body for most of my waking hours on coffee and soft drinks.

I mean, seriously, you never saw anyone who could drink coffee and Dr. Peppers the way I could. I lived in New Orleans in those days and taught at a ritzy prep school, and I'd have a minimum of six cups of New Orleans coffee with chicory and two packets of sugar every day of my life. Adding insult to injury, in the afternoons, I'd have a Dr. Pepper or two or three.

If you've been to New Orleans, you know the coffee there, just like the food, is intense. You can practically run a knife through a cup of New Orleans' coffee and see the track in the surface—like dragging a fork over the top of a newly iced cake. That's how strong the natives like their coffee in the Big Easy.

And I liked it too because it gave me remarkable energy for teaching English. I was a ball of fire, a live wire, a hot potato, a teacher known for his enthusiasm. The trouble was, after every class, I'd need another jolt of coffee or a Dr. Pepper to maintain that constant surge of energy.

Yeah, I'd down coffee until noon and then sip Dr. P's until school ended.

You see, in those days, I didn't have the natural, God-given, steady flow of energy I'm blessed with today because of my diet and lifestyle. The natural energy I enjoy today allows me to sit at my desk before dawn to write a daily health tip for twenty-one straight days when we did the contract challenge on the Internet, while also maintaining a huge web site and finishing the final desktop publishing revisions of a major cookbook. I'll also have the energy this afternoon to run a few miles before making dinner for my family. Hallelujah!

No sir. The energy I had in those days in New Orleans surged like an elevator out of control—up and down, up and down—jerk and stop—jerk and stop—and by the end of the day I looked as strung out as a clothes line made of barbed wire.

You'd have thought I needed Ritalin by the final bell at school.

Looking back on this period when I contributed so mightily to the weight and health problems that would hit me a few years later, I shudder.

You see I was flooding my body with sugar and caffeine, which, according to what we teach at Hallelujah Acres, are two very harmful substances.

Hey, wait, Chet, scientific studies prove that sugar and caffeine and alcohol in moderation are harmless. Don't you watch the nightly news?

I can hear someone out there muttering the above, and I reply, "I agree. If you do a search on Medline, sure enough, you can find scientific studies that 'prove' these poisons are harmless."

If you dig deeply enough, though, you can also find out who funded these studies.

Well, here at Hallelujah Acres we don't need hundred thousand dollar studies to prove to us that coffee and sugar are bad.

You see, we rely on common sense.

If you don't think coffee is bad for you, WHY do you feel so awful when you don't drink it for a few hours? Why do you get tremendous headaches when you try to stop drinking it altogether? Why do you need it to get started in the morning?

I'll tell you why.

Because coffee (and soft drinks and a host of other processed "foods") contain caffeine, which is an addictive drug—a powerful stimulant.

When you put any addictive drug in your body you're killing cells right and left. Common sense and even a little awareness of how the body works reveals to a thinking person that anything that gives you the jolt that coffee gives can't be good.

We deplore the use of heroin and other addictive drugs in our society and put people in jail for life for selling them.

And yet we have "scientific research" telling and "proving" to us that coffee and caffeine are "good" for us.

Baloney! Don't you see something wrong with the thinking here?

Continuing with our society's swallowing of another Big Lie, most soft drinks contain something like eleven teaspoons of sugar, and yet some modern research "studies" supposedly "prove" that sugar doesn't cause hyperactivity.

Gimme a break. I stand before you as a teacher with 25 year's experience in the classroom and shout, "Nonsense!" Ask teachers you know if sugar makes kids hyperactive and they'll tell you the same thing I'm telling you.

Friends, the soft drink industry has its tentacles wrapped around our schools, and this octopus without a conscience is squeezing the health right out of our children. As for the "artifical sweetners, the less said about those unnatural substances, the better.

Why are so many kids diagnosed as being hyperactive or ADD these days? Why are so many of our young people taking Ritalin?

At the schools where I used to teach, the faculty actually had medication breaks in some classes so all the students could take their Ritalin at the same time.

Walk around the campus and guess who you'd see chugging soft drinks between classes and on breaks? Just about every kid in school. And just about every faculty member to boot. Oh yeah, we had soda machines to help "raise activity funds."

At what cost? At what cost?

Well, anyway, you've caught me spurring my high horse even harder than usual, so let me dismount and just remind you that men, women, and children can NOT build superior health if they continue to drink soft drinks or coffee.

Period.

One final thought on this: As an experiment, get a meat–eating friend to save you a chicken bone and then drop that chicken bone in a glass of coke and let it stand overnight. See what kind of shape the bone is in the next morning. I strongly suspect you won't believe sugar and phosphoric acid are good for you after seeing what's left of that bone.

A few quick words about distilled water. We teach that distilled water is the best water to put in the body because it's the purest water available (outside of that found in fruits and vegetables, of course). As a next best alternative, we would recommend water that had been treated by reverse osmosis or a highly–rated filtering system.

Okay, enough about liquids.

Time for a recipe or two from Rhonda Malkmus' fabulous recipe book (see page 101 for details):

• • •

Cucumber Dressing
1 large cucumber
1 Tbsp. fresh lemon juice
1 green onion including top
2 Tbsp. dehydrated onion flakes
1/2 cup toasted sunflower seeds
1/2 tsp. Bragg Liquid Aminos (optional)

If the cucumber is not organic, peel it. If it is organic, some of the skin may be left on. Blend all ingredients until smooth and creamy. If a thinner dressing is desired, add distilled water.

• • •

Herb Lemon Dressing
1/3 cup lemon juice
1/3 cup honey
1 garlic clove
1/2 tsp. basil
1/3 cup distilled water
1 Tbsp. minced onion
1 tsp. oregano
1 Tbsp. Bragg Liquid Aminos (optional)

Mince garlic clove and onion and combine with liquids. Add herbs and allow to sit several hours for the flavors to combine.

• • •

Okie dokie, that does it for Day Five.

We'll be done with our first week before we know it, and I hope you're feeling as terrific on Day Five as I am.

Day Six of Our Twenty–One Days to Health the Hallelujah Diet Way

Good morning, fellow Hallelujah Health Seekers.

I'm going to devote today's letter to a few great letters that came in when I did the contract challenge on the Internet in January of 1998. Here are results reported after five days on the Hallelujah Diet. I've edited out questions and personal parts but have left in the best of the rest. Enjoy.

• • •

I've checked my scales and WOW! I've reduced my weight by five pounds already, and feeling tremendously ENERGETIC and excited about my energy. Can't keep the grin off my face! Also enjoying the feeling of not being overly full, not being bogged down with sugar and heaviness of extra unwanted unhealthy foods that make me feel a body feeling that I can only describe as 'THICK.'

Now, for a suggestion for one of your day letters. How about writing a real convicting letter for us to read that explains in detail what SUGAR does to our systems/body/mind/attitudes? I'd really like to read that, as I can certainly give up meat, give up white flour, even drink just vegetable juices and distilled water, but when you ask me to give up SUGAR? Whoa! Now, THAT's a hard one. I just love those jelly donuts, love those cookies, cakes, yum yum. I need a real convincing few paragraphs to give me the strength to have that self discipline when someone passes the dessert plate.

• • •

A pastor friend gave me a copy of Rev. Malkmus's first book—I read it straight through. Then I bought his second book last spring and started the Hallelujah Diet. I also purchased the seminar video. Got on Barleygreen & Herbal Fiberblend. You know what happened? I lost 47 pounds and really felt great. But as a pastor I got sidetracked last summer with nine weddings. Nine rehearsal dinners, nine receptions, etc, etc, etc. Anyway, I began to cheat on my diet and backslide. Then Thanksgiving & Christmas & I could not get the motivation to get with the program. Even though I knew better. Last fall I regained 30 pounds. But, here's the great news: Since beginning the diet on Monday I HAVE LOST NINE POUNDS and I am already beginning to have more energy. It's only Friday and I can't imagine how much I'll lose in the next sixteen days and thereafter. Boy does it feel great to have energy again. Glory!

Thanks again for all your work in this fantastic project. I want to become a health minister and get down for the training. Hope to meet you then.

• • •

Okay, it's Chet again, and I'm going to shut Day Six down with a recipe from Rhonda Malkmus and a wonderful little story that I hope will leave you laughing.

Almost everybody always wants to know how to deal with a sweet tooth healthfully. Here's a recipe that should fill that need in spades.

• • •

Frozen Raw Birthday Cake
submitted by Gracie Gordon
> 1 Bunt Cake Pan
> 16 oz. of dried organic figs, soaked overnight in distilled water*
> 16 oz. of dried pitted organic dates, soaked overnight in distilled water*
> 12 oz. bag of organic almonds
> 2 big bunches fully ripe bananas (organic if possible)

* Soak fruit in separate bowls. The water level for soaking is about half full. Do not cover the dried fruits completely.

Remove stems from soaked figs, puree figs and set aside. Puree dates put in separate bowl, chop almonds in food processor or blender and set aside in its own container. Peel and puree the bananas in a blender or food processor.

To Build the Cake

Place almonds in the bottom of the mold; 2nd layer, pureed figs; 3rd layer almonds; 4th layer pureed bananas, almonds, dates, almond, figs or whatever order you desire. Almonds should be the first layer and end with dates or figs the last layer. Cover and freeze overnight.

To Serve

Remove from the freezer, place upside down on a plate and allow to sit a few minutes until thawed enough to release from the pan. Can be carefully set in warm water just long enough to release the cake, being very careful not to get water in the cake.

This cake has so many possibilities. Use strawberries and blueberries for a beautiful, healthy Fourth of July cake. Any of your favorite fruits can be used to make a new family tradition.

• • •

Laughter truly is the best medicine, and here's something to tickle your funny bone that almost put me on the floor when I received it in my e–mail:

• • •

The Missionary's Horse

A man has been lost and walking in the desert for about two weeks.

One hot day (of course, they're all hot), he comes to the home of a missionary. Tired and weak, he crawls up to the house and collapses on the doorstep. The missionary takes him in and nurses him back to health. Feeling better, the man asks the missionary for directions to the nearest town. The missionary tells him that he must borrow the horse to make it. He says, "However, there is a special thing about this horse. You have to say 'Thank God' to make it go and 'Amen' to make it stop."

Now anxious to get to town, the man says, "Sure, OK," and he gets on the horse. He says, "Thank God," and the horse starts walking. A bit later he says louder, "Thank God, thank God," and the horse starts trotting. Feeling really brave, the man say, "Thank God! Thank God! THANK GOD!" and the horse is soon up to a full run!

About then he realizes he's heading for a huge cliff edge, and he yells, "Whoa!" but the horse doesn't even slow! The cliff edge is coming up REAL QUICK and he's doing everything he can to make the horse stop. "Whoa, stop, hold on!" Finally he remembers; "AMEN!"

The horse stops four inches from the cliff, almost throwing him over its head. The man, panting and heart racing, wipes the sweat from his face and leans back in the saddle.

"Oh!" he says, gasping for air, "Thank God."

• • •

Hang in there. Week One is almost over, and the best is yet to come.

Day Seven of Our Twenty–One Days to Health the Hallelujah Diet Way

Good morning, fellow Hallelujah Health Seekers.

We're at the end of our first week already, and if you're feeling as good as many of the people on our program feel after seven days, then you're whistling "Dixie" and vibrating like a downed power line—and everybody else in your house is still asleep while you're up and at it.

It's about a quarter to seven on a Sunday morning as I write these words, and I've been up and at it for a bit, answering more of the wonderful e–mail that *pours* in every day of the week from people here in America as well as around the world. While answering the mail, I got to thinking about some time I spent recently with Dr. Malkmus.

On a Saturday in January, I went hiking with Dr. Malkmus on his beautiful property in the mountains north of Shelby, North Carolina, and as we walked we continually remarked on the beauty and wonders of God's creation.

We also talked about how the human body is so like the forests—all around us we saw plants and trees stripped of leaves, and yet, at the same time, we saw new growth everywhere.

One tree in particular amazed me. It grows directly above a natural spring— indeed the spring literally flows from where the huge old tree bursts from the earth.

This tree must be twelve feet in diameter at its base, and it towers above the other trees. How appropriate and how true to God's laws of nature that a constant supply of nutrients and water from the earth would make this tree the strongest and healthiest one in the forest.

Since you're on the 21–day contract you too now have the knowledge to live your life like this tree—you too can tap into the marvelous self–healing nature built into us by God and you can fuel your body with real food instead of processed junk.

All of us on this program can cleanse our body/temples.

We too can stand taller than the other trees in the forest.

And then we can share our knowledge so all the people in the sick and suffering concrete jungles of the cities of the earth can join us in leading healthy, happy, service–filled lives.

All right.

Before I share with you a few great letters that show the benefits of the Hallelujah Diet, let's first have a recipe. Here's one from Rhonda Malkmus' *Recipes for Life… from God's Garden* (see page 101) that's terrific for getting the all–important, cell–building green vegetation into your diet.

• • •

Mixed Greens with Apples

1 cup of spinach
1 large Granny Smith apple
1 cup of kale
1 cup of leaf lettuce
1 cup of Swiss chard or other greens of choice

Tear greens into bite–sized pieces. Peel and dice apple into small pieces. Mix well. Top with Poppy Seed Dressing (see below).

• • •

Poppy Seed Dressing

4 Tbsp. fresh lemon juice
4 Tbsp. fresh orange juice
1/2 cup soaked almonds
2 Tbsp. green onion
1/2 tsp. paprika
2 Tbsp. poppy seeds

Place almonds in a bowl, cover with distilled water, and soak overnight. Drain and place all ingredients in blender except poppy seeds. Blend until desired consistency is reached, adding distilled water if needed. Stir poppy seeds in by hand before serving.

• • •

Now that you know how to make a mixed greens with apple salad, let's turn to some letters I want to share with you this beautiful morning.

The first letter provides a long list of details about the dangers of processed sugar:

• • •

Dear Chet:

In response to the sugar question. Sugar is a drug. Sugar is additive. Sugar can and does affect the body in many ways. The following information comes from Nancy Appleton, M.D. who wrote, "Lick the Sugar Habit."

Sugar can:
- *suppress the immune system (three soft drinks will wipe out the immune system for the day);*
- *upset the minerals in the body;*
- *cause hyperactivity, anxiety, difficulty concentrating;*
- *produce a significant rise in triglycerides;*
- *cause reduction in defense against bacterial infection;*
- *cause kidney damage;*
- *reduce high density lipoproteins;*
- *lead to chromium deficiency;*

- *lead to cancer of the breast, ovaries, intestines, prostate, and rectum;*
- *increase fasting levels of glucose and insulin;*
- *cause copper deficiency;*
- *interfere with absorption of calcium and magnesium;*
- *weaken eyesight;*
- *raise the level of neurotransmitters called serotonin;*
- *cause hypoglycemia;*
- *produce an acidic stomach;*
- *cause aging, arthritis, asthma, candida, gallstones, appendicitis, heart disease, multiple sclerosis, hemorrhoids, varicose veins, and periodontal disease;*
- *increase cholesterol, migraine headaches, interferes with the absorption of protein;*
- *cause toxemia during pregnancy;*
- *impair the structure of DNA;*
- *cause cataracts, emphysema, atherosclerosis;*
- *can cause free radicals in the bloodstream;*
- *and it can cause hunger pains and overeating.*

These are only some of the side effects of eating sugar.

Chet, I know you're busy so I thought I would help you out on this one.

I'm sure that sugar (except from fruit and veggies) is one of the drugs that we should avoid. Although we use honey, we try to use it sparingly.

New Years Eve someone offered us some brownies. I ate two brownies and couldn't stop. I then ate a chocolate chip cookie, an ice cream bar, and a honey bun roll.

That night I was totally depressed. My husband and I got into a big fight. The next day I looked back at what I had eaten and it was Sugar.

I guess that's what you would call a doubleblind study. I won't be doing that again.

• • •

This second letter was one of my favorites during the 21–day contract challenge on the Internet in January of 1998:

• • •

Chet:

Really appreciate all your work with the 21–day contract letters. They've been very helpful and inspiring. I've been fighting the Hallelujah Diet because I've always been a "picky" eater and a lot of things I just don't like, including a lot of fruits and vegetables. I knew the Hallelujah Diet made sense but just wasn't sure I could handle it.

Your three week challenge was a great nudge in the right direction. The first day I thought I might be starving to death and about half of the second day I was still feeling doubtful that I could survive on salad and raw veggies.

By the second evening, though, I was starting to calm down a bit and realized that I could survive on this. By Day Three the hunger pains subsided. I really appreciate you sharing your menu, and a friend of mine that has been on the Hallelujah Diet for several months has also been real helpful about advising me what was "good" or "legal."

I have always had a HUGE sweet tooth and consumed some form of candy or cookie every day. I used to think it was a real milestone to go a day with no candy. I craved it terribly. I am truly amazed and shocked that since starting this healthy way of eating and not allowing myself to cheat even a little bit that the craving has stopped.

Not to say I don't think I might like something sweet, but it's not that serious craving, gotta have it, kind of feeling. Wow! I never thought I'd see the day when that happened.

I'm thrilled to report that as of this morning I have lost five pounds and I look forward to losing more as I make this healthy way of eating MY way of eating. Praise the Lord for you and all those trying to help others learn about the importance of eating healthy!

• • •

Dear Chet:

After six great days on this I feel fantastic—clean and with a lot of energy. I am never hungry, which is an absolute miracle for me! The biggest plus, though, is that I have not been controlled by food and thoughts of food this week—it has really been a freeing experience!

I have tried things I never would have dreamt of trying without your example. The first one that comes to mind is the blended salad. I love it! I can add veggies I usually have a hard time eating raw (like broccoli) and then it's a cinch to eat. I really enjoy experimenting with it and trying different things. It's great with a little hummus or a little baba ganoush or just garlic and lemon with the avocado! I didn't find it difficult to make either—it was actually fun shoving everything in there with the celery stalk! Thanks!

I want to second the request for more info on the evils of sugar. I am a sugar addict! I can't stop if I have just a little. The one thing that helps me stay away from it is knowing what it does to my immune system! And this is a wonderful time for us to be eating so healthy—flu season.

• • •

Chet:

I don't know where to begin as to what God has done in my life this past week. I suffer from what the doctors call Fibromyalgia. I also have disc problems in my lower back. I began this diet about one month ago halfheartedly. I took meat, most fats, and salts out of my diet and cut back on my sugar intake. At the time I started the diet I was taking seven different prescriptions including ones with codeine. These were to help me sleep, relieve pain, and to help with the total body fatigue.

In the past few years I have been unable to clean the house or care for my family the way I would like to. I have this past year been forced to use a cane because of my leg. That was in the past since my contract which I am following 98%. Now I clean my own home. I am able to stand and cook at the end of the day instead of putting up my swollen legs.

Last night after a full day with my children (whom I home school) I went grocery shopping. In the past I would have had to take a nap first. I am no longer taking two of my pain medications and for the first time in a year I am not taking any codeine. Today I am planning to take a walk with my husband (who is also on the contract with me). He said only for twenty–one days, but since seeing my progress has decided to make it a lifestyle change. I thank my Heavenly Father for showing such loving care for me and bringing this diet to my attention. It is proof once more that the Bible is the one and only, and the final authority.

• • •

Dear Chet:

Day Five, 6 p.m—Got the neatest message from my body today, talking spinach talk. I was tired, cranky & hungry at five o'clock, barely dragging. Managed to get supper on the table for family & friends, then finally collapsed into my chair with a bowl of fresh spinach leaves from a supermarket bag.

How do you like my spinach salad recipe? "1) buy bag, 2) open bag, 3) eat green leaves. Fork optional." Well, I did add a splash of bottled vinaigrette. A piquant bit of whimsy.

About the time I finished chewing the leaves, I realized my feet didn't hurt anymore! Neither did my back. And my head felt as good as it did at lunchtime when I was having my "snuff." (As a little kid I envied my grandma's snuff. I knew she got pleasure from it, but the taste—yuck!) Today, on a lark, I snuffed some Barleygreen. One tsp. dry powder in lower lip. Drink a glass of water before 'cause you can't after. THEN...

I worked non–stop for the next five hours. Scrubbing, cleaning, reorganizing, dumping clutter, preparing company supper, arranging cut flowers, dismantling the kitchen desk and converting it into a raw–food preparation center: cutting board, Champion juicer, food dehydrator, processor, blender, etc. Didn't even pause to change from dress shoes to jogging shoes (a mistake). Volunteered to pick up a teenage friend at 5 PM and run some errands. Ran out of steam half way home. Man, was I tired and grumpy. Didn't realize I had just burned up all my food energy until it came springing back when I ate the spinach.

Message? "Fresh, raw spinach is a fatigue chaser." And a grump–buster. And the energy is fresher. Stronger, clearer, calmer. Not a tad scrambled by the drying process in green juice powder.

How do I know for sure? Immediately after the spinach salad, I thought I was still hungry (didn't wait 15 minutes) and took a bite of chili. Within minutes I got that sinking feeling as if my energy was being drained away (actually, the blood being drawn down to my stomach to digest meat). As soon as I put two and two together, I dashed to the refrigerator, grabbed a fist full of spinach leaves and stuffed them in my mouth. As I chewed it I began feeling clear–headed again.

Cause & effect. Simple, direct, and so–ooo obvious. Precursor to the scientific method. Any scientist could replicate the experiment if he'd been on 100% raw long enough to flush the gunk out of his analytic organ. Especially if he is hypoglycemic & pre–diabetic like me and gets drowsy after eating most cooked foods.

Now it's 4 a.m. Since supper, I have attacked the bedroom clutter and can report that the floor is visible again, after weeks of Christmas chaos; read & processed 60 e–mail messages and updated my 21–day contract journal which you are reading right now.

Now it's 4:08 a.m., and finally, I'm yawning.

• • •

Do you now see why everyone at Hallelujah Acres loves what they're doing? Can you imagine how I feel every day of my life when I get to read mail like this as soon as I log onto the Internet? Can you imagine how Dr. Malkmus feels when he sits down and reads not only the e–mails I share with him but literally hundreds of other letters like these that arrive in the regular mail every week of the year?

My friend, our program works wonders for so many people.

Hallelujah.

Tomorrow we begin Week Two, and I promise you it will be the best one yet. See you then.

Day Eight of Our Twenty–One Days to Health the Hallelujah Diet Way

Good morning, fellow Hallelujah Health Seeker.

Today you and I begin our second week of our *Twenty–One Days to Health the Hallelujah Diet Way.*

And to get it off to a quick start, I want to say a few words about the good things you can expect during the next two weeks.

Obviously, we are all different so not everyone will enjoy all of the following benefits we hear about every day at Hallelujah Acres, but many will experience at least some of these positive changes. Below find listed a few major benefits people report after they've been on the Hallelujah Diet for a few weeks:

Continued weight loss until the body reaches its ideal weight

I personally went from 200 lbs. to 145 lbs. in about three months. Although my weight has fluctuated as much as ten pounds during the past five years, I don't seem to be normal in this respect since most people who get on the diet and stay on the diet pretty much remain at their ideal weight.

Less need for sleep

I used to require eight to ten hours, even on a natural vegetarian diet. When I began the Hallelujah Diet and added Barleygreen and carrot juice to my routine, my sleep needs went down dramatically. These days I feel really good on five to seven hours of sleep a night.

Deeper and more refreshing sleep

I've always been a light sleeper and that's still true. A fly batting against a light bulb can wake me up, and I used to have a terrible time getting back to sleep. These days, if I haven't yet gotten the sleep I need for a particular night, even if a noise or something wakes me up, I'll zoom right back to Dreamland.

More energy

Most people who get on the Hallelujah Diet just can't believe how their energy increases as they continue to practice the diet. Dr. Malkmus is a human dynamo, for example, and he maintains a work schedule that would drop most people in their tracks. Additionally, even though he turned 64 in 1998, he can still scurry up a mountain faster than athletes half his age.

Less hunger

In my SAD days, I could sit down and eat a large Dominos pizza, drink a quart of coke, and then be nibbling on a bag of corn chips an hour later. I was always hungry. Of course I now know that was because I wasn't giving my body anything with any nutrition in it. Once you get the nutrient flood of the Hallelujah Diet, however, you'll probably note that you require less and less food as time goes by.

Diminished body odor

After most people finish detoxing, they find they no longer have any body odor and can then say good–bye to underarm deodorants, breath mints, and scented oils and aftershaves.

Better ability to sweat

Our skin serves as our largest organ of elimination, and the longer you practice the Hallelujah Lifestyle, the easier you'll break into a sweat. This may sound yucky if you dine a lot with the Vanderbilts, but for most of us perspiring is a good thing because the more you sweat, the more your body can eliminate toxins and other junk that it doesn't want to store inside tissue, muscles, organs, and so on.

Heightened awareness

Just about everyone who's been on the diet for a few months will tell you that their senses improve dramatically. The sense of taste becomes so acute that you will begin to enjoy the subtle flavors of bland veggies like carrots. The sense of smell becomes so keen that you'll have trouble standing close to someone who wears perfume or aftershave. The sense of sight improves, and some people actually stop wearing glasses. The sense of touch gets better, and you really do get to the point where you can hear a pin drop.

Increased clarity of mind

Those days of muddled thinking become a thing of the past. You can work calculus problems that puzzled Einstein; you can write symphonies that left Bach pulling his hair out, and you can play Jeopardy with the best of them. Well, maybe things don't get quite that good, but you will find that you think a whole lot better than you did on the SAD.

Fewer mood swings

This is one of my favorites since I used to have more than my share of blue periods before I changed my diet. These days I'm so happy and positive almost all the time that some people find me annoying. Many people who suffered depression report that they get off all medication after being on the Hallelujah Diet for various periods of time.

Better ability to deal with stress

When you're physically, mentally, and emotionally at your best, you can handle the trials and tribulations of 20th century life in the fast lane a lot easier than when you were toxic, overweight, and out of shape. Little things that used to drive you nuts you'll accept with a grin after you've been on the Hallelujah Diet for a few months.

Fewer colds and flus

Many people on the Hallelujah Diet who have thoroughly detoxed and who follow the diet carefully, exercise each day, keep their stress levels down, and so on find that they just plain don't get sick at all anymore. I haven't had to miss work for going on two years now, and Dr. Malkmus can say the same thing—but for over twenty years. Truly, you don't have to be sick.

Immunity from chronic disease

Those who start the program young enough may well never have to deal with any of the mid–life (or earlier) diseases that many people are now dealing with. With the Hallelujah Diet, God's self–healing immune system works the way it was designed to work, and consequently most people who practice the whole program just plain won't get sick and will probably never experience the diseases that are ruining the quality of life of so many senior citizens today.

Increased spirituality

I've saved what I personally consider the best for last. Since I've been on the Hallelujah Diet, my spiritual growth has been a constant source of joy. My faith has deepened, and my connection with God has intensified to the point where it's with me every second of my life. I have a desire to serve others that I lacked the first 45 years of my life. I see God's hand everywhere and in everything. Hallelujah!

Are the above all the benefits that come from living life the Hallelujah Way?

Not at all. There are many others, but these represent the ones that have impacted most people the most. And, just think, most people, over time, can experience these benefits even if they're ill when they start.

Okay, let's turn to one more of the wonderful letters I received during the Internet 21–day contract challenge:

• • •

Dear Chet:

Just wanted you to know that I'm doing OK with my weight now… I'm eating a large baked potato with my evening meals and that seems to really help. Sometimes I'll have my buckwheat noodles at noon with my salad. By the way, they are delicious. They have a nice flavor and can be found in the Chinese or Asian section of your supermarket. As for my health, I'm thinking clearer, have much more energy, stay up till 10:00 p.m. and have much less muscle pain. This is a great diet. While family members take naps, I'm now the one doing the errands, giving rides, etc. because I have so much more energy!

• • •

About this time in the contract, many people start hungering for bread, so let me provide a good recipe from Rhonda Malkmus' *Recipes for Life… from God's Garden.*

• • •

Honey Nut Oatmeal Bread
submitted by Kay Frost
    1 1/3 cups distilled water
    1/4 cup honey
    1 cup whole wheat flour
    2 1/2 tsp. yeast
    2 tbsp. unsweetened applesauce
    1 cup rolled oats
    2 cups bread flour
    2/3 cups walnuts

Place all ingredients in a bread machine except walnuts. Turn machine on to the Sweet Bread setting. Chop walnuts. At the beep, add the walnuts and continue baking until the machine shuts off.

• • •

Okay, that wraps it up for Day Eight. I hope you're sharing the good news of the Hallelujah Diet with friends, relatives, acquaintances, and people at work because the more of us who spread the health message, the quicker we can help to end the disease and suffering that's impacting so many lives in our country and around the world.

See you tomorrow.

Day Nine of Our Twenty–One Days to Health the Hallelujah Diet Way

Good morning, fellow Hallelujah Health Seeker.

You're reading your Day Nine Newsletter from a guy who turned a half century old today.

Whoa. Holy moly. Wow!

I mean, seriously, I never in a zillion years thought I'd charge into my fifth decade of life and feel like I'd just turned 18.

In fact, up until five years ago, I dreaded turning fifty because I had been taught that was when you really started falling apart; that fifty was when you prepared yourself for the mid–life illness that would either take you down completely or else leave you a shadow of your former self; that fifty was the beginning of the end.

What baloney! What nonsense. What hooey!

You see, thanks to living by God's natural laws, today I honestly feel better than I felt when I was 18.

Yeah, better.

I got tired when I was 18. It's a rare day when I get tired here at 50.

As the famous old James Brown classic puts it, "I feel good!"

Here I am fifty years old, bouncing out of bed every day of the week and chomping at the bit to do what has become my life's work: to spread the "You don't have to be sick" message to anyone who will turn even half an ear to listen to it.

Here I am fifty years old, writing like a maniac for sometimes ten hours a day and then getting home and feeling so good I actually want to go outside and jog for two or three or four miles.

Here I am fifty years old, finishing my run and still feeling so good that now I want to go into the garage to lift weights for another twenty minutes of exercise.

Here I am fifty years old, eager every evening after exercising to go into the kitchen and make a big ole glass of carrot/apple/celery/lettuce juice that I'll sip and enjoy the way most people enjoy fine wines.

Here I am fifty years old and not grumpy because I have to clean the juicer. Stuff like that rarely makes me grouchy anymore. Amazing.

Here I am fifty years old, having a lot of fun preparing a supper that consists of a huge tub of green lettuce and chopped veggies followed by a plate of rice with some lightly steamed veggies on top of it.

Here I am fifty years old, enjoying the give and take of a family dinner with two teenage sons and my first wife, who I still find fascinating after almost 26 years of marriage.

Let's do a quick flashback to last evening, the night before I turned fifty:

Here I am the night before my birthday, getting a kick out of Number Two

Son rubbing it in like hand lotion: "Hey, Dad, you're going to be FIFTY years old tomorrow."

Here I am reminding Number Two Son I can still take him outside and run him right into the dirt any day of the week. (Number One Son has the kindness not to mention that he can now take me outside any day of the week and run me right into the dirt, but from the grin on his face I can see he's tempted to point it out.)

Here I am fifty years old, done with dinner and clean–up and feeling light and energetic and ready to plop down on the couch to read Herbert Shelton or Paul Bragg or Norman Walker or George Malkmus or another of the great alternative health movement writers for an hour or two.

Here I am fifty years old, around ten p.m., meditating, at total peace, silently and wondrously in touch with God.

Here I am fifty years old, snuggling under the covers and falling asleep almost instantly.

Here I am, fifty years old, as happy and healthy and content as I've ever been in my life.

You know, friends, I sat down this morning to write an entirely different Day Nine tip and the above just flowed out of me like juice from a Green Power juicer, and I decided to share these thoughts with you, not to brag about myself but to document what can happen to a very normal, typical person who was brought up as most of us are brought up on the Standard American Diet, believing the Standard American Lie about the medical profession offering our only hope for healthy lives.

You see, when I started to fall apart at age 44, unwilling to follow the medical route that has basically ruined the health of my parents and almost ruined the health of my wife, I decided to go the nutritional lifestyle route instead.

I tried a two–week experiment very similar to what we're doing together for three weeks right now, and I've never looked back.

Today, I'm so happy to have the chance to share this wonder in my life with you, someone who made the same decision—to follow God's way to health instead of man's way.

My wish for you on this celebration of my first half century of life is that you take charge of your health and thus feel as good as I do on your 40th or 50th or 60th or 70th or 80th or 90th birthday.

How about a quick look at a good letter from a fellow Hallelujah Health Seeker:

• • •

I tried doing the Hallelujah Diet off and on, but never stuck with it. A close friend of mine was put on Dr. Atkins diet (lots of meat and eggs, NO fruit!) and I tried that for a week or so just to lose weight, but every time I ate I felt guilty because I knew this wasn't healthy! I knew I had to go on the Hallelujah Diet, and your letter of encouragement to try it for 21 days was what got me started.

I have been on it for a week and have been reading all these wonderful letters you've been passing on. I kept thinking WHY don't I have a wonder story to tell? Sure, I feel good, and I don't wake up during the night with a stomach ache thinking "I'm never going to eat again!" but that didn't seem like a wonder story to me. I thought, "Why don't I have a TON of energy?" But I know it's because I haven't been exercising along with the diet. This morning I thought, "Why don't I wake up with a burst of energy?" but I knew it was because I stayed up til 11:45 p.m last night! After I got up and got going, my mind cleared, and THEN it hit me!

I have had a cold virus for two months. I have been coughing my head off much of that time. Couldn't function without cough drops. A day or two after I began the Hallelujah Diet, I began again with a constant runny nose, and thought "Oh great! Here I go again!" But guess what! This morning I realized MY COLD IS GONE! I am not coughing, I don't have a runny nose! Oh wow! I DO have a wonder story!" Just had to share it with you!

• • •

Now, if that letter's not inspiring, I'll eat my sweat socks after jogging five miles. Yuck to the max.

Speaking of eating, please try this great live food recipe from Rhonda Malkmus:

• • •

Raw Stuffed Peppers

  1 red bell pepper for each person
  1 large avocado
  2 scallions
  2 celery stalks
  2 tomatoes
  1/2 cup grated cabbage

Wash pepper, remove top, ribs, and seeds. Set aside. Grate cabbage, finely chop celery, dice tomatoes, chop scallions, mash the avocado, combine all chopped vegetables and stuff pepper.

• • •

Okay, that wraps it up for Day Nine. I hope you're also sharing the good news with friends, relatives, acquaintances, and people at work because the more of us who spread the health message, the quicker we can help to end the disease and suffering that's impacting so many lives in our country and around the world. See you tomorrow.

Day Ten of Our Twenty–One Days to Health the Hallelujah Diet Way

Good morning, fellow Hallelujah Health Seeker.

With each passing day, we receive more and more wonderful testimonies of how the Hallelujah Diet is working in people's lives. I'm going to share several of those letters with you in a few moments, but first I want to remind you that you must have patience when you change your lifestyle and your way of eating.

I had several letters from individuals doing the 21–day contract on the Internet who experienced frustration because they weren't seeing the same wonderful results seen in the "good news" letters you read each day in this book.

Please remember that each person's body carries a different level of toxicity and each person's immune system functions at a different level of efficiency, and each person heals at a different speed.

The important and primary principal is that God graced our bodies with a self–healing mechanism.

Our bodies, when given the proper fuels and conditions, will always work toward ideal health.

The hard part is that most of us have lived and eaten poorly for most of our lives and consequently our immune systems are sluggish and inefficient.

Some immune systems reactivate like lightning slamming into a solitary oak tree, and these lucky folks quickly regain their energy, quickly have their minds clear up, and quickly start feeling great again.

Hallelujah for this.

Other folks who may have chronic diseases that have battered their immune systems for months or even years won't have the immediate and dramatic results. Instead, their improvements will come in increments.

This, of course, leads to frustration and thoughts of "Well, this diet doesn't work for me."

Although we don't claim that our program works for everyone, we are confident that just about everyone can reap at least some benefit from sticking with the Hallelujah Diet for a three–month period. Dr. Malkmus teaches that it takes at least three months for most people to be well on their way to a thorough detox and reactivation of the immune system.

But not everyone is going to heal 100% in three months or in six months or nine months or even a year. Some will heal in weeks; others will literally take years. Please remember that it took Dr. Malkmus a full twelve months on raw foods and carrot juice alone to heal his colon cancer. He didn't give up in a few weeks or a few months. He stuck with the Genesis 1:29 diet until he was well. He had faith in God's self–healing mechanism—he believed it would work if he provided his body with the right fuel and conditions.

And it did.

And it's still working today, more than twenty years later, as Dr. Malkmus remains the picture of health, thanks to the Hallelujah Diet.

But it didn't happen overnight.

So, if you're not progressing as rapidly as others on the contract, *please* do not despair or give up.

And remember also that best results come by working the entire program: diet, exercise, sunshine, peace of mind, good family relationships, and so on.

Please consider this: you've only been working the program for ten days, and if you feel even the slightest bit better after ten days, isn't that progress? Don't you have the patience to continue for another eleven days to see how you'll feel then?

If you haven't yet seen the results you're hoping for, I urge you to hang in there, to stick with the program for at least the duration of your contract.

God willing, you too will begin to see the improvements so many others are experiencing.

Okay, time for some more wonderful letters:

• • •

Chet:

I had been on thyroid medication for six years and was told it would be the rest of my life. But after 33 days on the Hallelujah Diet/Lifestyle, juicing carrots, (my husband and I juice approximately 50 pounds of carrots a week) and taking two–three tablespoons of Barleygreen a day, my doctor took me off the medication and told me that the kelp in the Barleygreen was the big help for my major improvement.

I should also say that I stopped all allergy shots and inhaler use and lost 25 pounds. And the reason we started this in March of 1996 was because of four surgeries (over three years) to remove melanoma from my husband that kept recurring every eight months. We are thankful beyond words to say that he has remained cancer–free for twenty–one months, as of Jan. 1, 1998.

We are now Health Ministers and Praise God for this program and believe in it 100%. I have tons of energy and we feel great. It is not easy, but neither were all the trips to Oklahoma City for surgery and treatments and checkups. Why would anyone go back to the world's way of eating when God's way is so superior?

We encourage the 90 day trial and challenge people to really be open to changes as they see for themselves that they don't have to be sick!

• • •

Dear Chet:

I have been on the Hallelujah Diet for a week now and am happy to say I have lost seven pounds and have more energy than I have had in a long time. I must tell you about how great your trampoline idea was. My daughter moved and left this little trampoline in my garage, so when I read your idea, I went and got that out, dusted it off and put it in my bedroom.

I am 60+ years old. The first time I got on it, I could only do about five jumps, but after four days I am up to 100 jumps and feel so good. I am enjoying the daily

letters and recipes you send. I am grateful to my daughter for telling me about you and the new way of eating. It does make me feel so much better. Keep up Gods' work.
Happy Birthday

• • •

Golly, I'm running out of space again already, but here's a quick recipe from Rhonda's cookbook for you to enjoy:

• • •

Sunshine Carrot Salad

3 cups carrot
1/2 cup organic raisins
1 Red Delicious apple
1 stalk of celery

Peel and grate apple and carrots and finely chop celery. Combine all ingredients above in a bowl and toss. Mix in the following dressing:

1 Red Delicious apple
2 cups grated carrots
1/2 cup almonds
fresh apple juice or distilled water

In a blender, chop 1/2 cup of almonds, add one Red Delicious apple, peeled and cored, and two cups of grated carrot. Blend until creamy. Add a small amount of distilled water or fresh apple juice to reach consistency desired.

• • •

Okay, that wraps it up for Day Ten.

Can you believe it? We're just about halfway through the contract already. Time sure flies when you're having fun, doesn't it?

Day Eleven of Our Twenty–One Days to Health the Hallelujah Diet Way

Good morning, fellow Hallelujah Health Seeker.

Pat yourself on the back, look yourself in the mirror, smile like the cat that swallowed the canary, and then dash outside and shout to the world, "I'm halfway through my 21–day contract. Hallelujah!"

Of course if you're shouting too loud, a crowd will gather around you, but that's okay. You can use this opportunity to share with them precisely what you're doing and why you're losing weight and feeling more energetic than you've felt in years.

Whoa, Chet, put on the brakes and rein in the horses—we're halfway there, not standing tall as we run into home after knocking the health ball clean out of Yankee Stadium.

Okay, okay, we'll save the big celebrating for Day Twenty–One, the day we actually complete the contract.

I'm looking back on my first eleven days of this contract with satisfaction, and I hope you are too. I've been tempted a couple of times, especially on my birthday when my wife kept asking me if I wanted a cake, but I managed to fight the good fight and went this year without eating three huge pieces of the usual wonderful–tasting cherry–chocolate cake concoction that always makes me grumpy and constipated the next day.

Golly—three huge pieces. Yep, I'm one of those all or nothing guys. When I'm working, I work. When I'm sleeping, I sleep. And when I'm eating cherry–chocolate cake with whipped cream icing, I'm not nibbling on celery.

But this year I said, "No thanks," and consequently I felt great the day after my 50th birthday instead of feeling like I'd just turned 109 after living all those years on the SAD (Standard American Diet).

Okay, enough warm–up—time for today's topic. Today I want to remind you once more that although we call our program the Hallelujah Diet, most of us on it think of it as a lifestyle rather than a diet.

Remember, the daily diet of juicing, predominently raw fruits and vegetables, some whole grained pastas and breads and cooked vegetables, and Barleygreen represents just part of our overall program to ultimate health.

As taught by the 19th and early 20th century health reformers from Sylvester Graham to Russell Thrall to John Tilden to Herbert Shelton to Paul Bragg, Dr. Malkmus also incorporates into his total lifestyle program several other important elements. For the sake of completeness, let me list them and comment briefly.

Diet

Ideally, humanity would thrive best on the Genesis 1:29 diet. But most of us don't live in ideal conditions, so we also include some cooked food for the evening meal because most people have a very difficult time eating all raw. We add carrot and vegetable juicing and Barleygreen several times a day to provide our deficient bodies with a literal flood of nutrients that most of us won't get in our supermarket foods.

Exercise

We teach that optimal health requires up to an hour's worth of aerobic exercise each day. We consider brisk walking the best of the best, though we encourage each individual to find the exercise that makes him/her the happiest. Other excellent aerobic exercises include rebounding, swimming, bicycling, jogging, and mud wrestling. (Just kidding—though, now that I think about it, wrestling does provide a fantastic workout. But instead of seizing some stranger off the street and throwing him down in a plowed field that just embraced a rain storm, why not grab a couple of your kids and challenge them to a wrestling match? Just be sure you're already in pretty good shape before you do this because 'rassling can quickly turn into anaerobic exercise and really gets the old ticker pumping in a hurry.)

Rest

Each of us absolutely requires a certain amount of sleep each night. Most of us are terribly sleep deficient because we lead crazy lives of working too hard for too many hours. And when we're not working, we're scurrying around like ants to the cookie jar going from one errand to another. And when we're not running around, too many of us are glued in front of the television set soaking up sports or movies or TV shows until it's way past our natural bed–time—sundown. If you want to achieve optimal health, you must get your sleep habits in order, and you should go to bed early enough so you'll wake up naturally in the morning without grogginess or without having an alarm blast you into consciousness.

Prayer or Meditation

You must spend some time developing your spirituality each day. We are physical, mental, emotional, and spiritual beings, and if we neglect any of these parts of ourselves we can't achieve optimal health. If you don't spend at least twenty minutes a day in prayer, Bible study, meditation, or some other form of communion with God, I highly recommend that you add this to your daily routine. I consider my silent time each night the crowning blessing to a day thoroughly well–lived.

Emotional Poise

Most of us spend our lives on emotional roller coasters, pulling ourselves up the initial stretch when we get out of bed in the morning and then zooming up and down, up and down, as we deal with the various stresses of the day. To attain optimal health, we have to train ourselves to stay emotionally balanced—if we don't, our bodies are constantly flooded with adrenaline and other hormones that upset equilibrium.

Clean Air and Clean Water

These factors are pretty self–explanatory. If we're breathing dirty air and drinking water polluted with chlorine, fluoride, heavy metals, parasites, and Lord knows what else, we're putting foreign substances in that the body must then either store or excrete. So we teach that the ideal is to live in areas as unpolluted as possible and to drink freshly extracted vegetable juices and distilled water only.

Sunshine

If you're not getting outside in the sun once in a while, you're never going to achieve optimal health because your body needs sunshine. Not only for Vitamin D but for other reasons nobody has yet identified. Without sounding too strange, all I can tell you is that when I'm out in the sun, I feel like a battery being recharged from a cross country power line. I didn't feel this way five years ago when I first started doing everything I could to get at least twenty minutes of sun on my bod every day, but I sure do now. As our bodies purify, we become more sensitive not only to the wonderful natural flavors of fresh foods, but we also become more sensitive to the life–giving powers of the sun. When I lived in Florida and Louisiana, I got out in the sun almost every single day, and I was usually out in it in a pair of jogging shorts and shoes and nothing else. Now that we're undergoing winter in North Carolina, I'm not getting that daily sun, and I miss it. I can't tell you how much I look forward to spring and the return of the sun.

Happy Relationships

Finally, for optimal health you need to be a loving person who accepts all people for who and what they are. You need to develop loving attitudes toward everyone in your life, including family members, relatives, friends, and acquaintances. If you're not happy with other people, you're not going to be happy with yourself. Time spent with loved ones is the most important time of all.

Okay, there you have it—the Hallelujah Lifestyle in a nutshell. If you practice all of the above and get these factors worked into your daily routine, you have the best chance of attaining optimal health.

Will you be able to do all of the above every day? Maybe—if you're retired or independently wealthy and don't have to earn a living. But most of us don't live in this kind of world, so we have to do the best we can.

And that's the key to this, my friend: do the best you can each day.

Be patient and loving with yourself and strive for gradual improvements. Try to work the diet and exercise every day and then add in the others as you can—it sounds intimidating at first, but it can be done, believe me.

And the results in a few short months will hopefully have you shouting from the rooftop with your new–found energy and love of life.

Hallelujah!

I was rather long–winded today and took up most of the space, so I'll close my yap and drop in a couple of good letters from fellow contract brothers and sisters:

• • •

Chet:

Loved your letter. It made me feel good just reading it. I turned 50 in November. But I wasn't thinking the same thoughts you were. My thoughts were, "Gee, I'm too young to feel this old!" I was a bit depressed, to say the least.

But today is a new day and I have received a wonderful gift! I woke up feeling full of energy, my legs don't feel as if I'm carrying around sand bags and I feel very optimistic.

Praise God for helping me to find your web site. I have been truly blessed. Miracles do happen.

• • •

Dear Chet:

My wife Mary signed up on the 21–day contract; however, there are now four in our family who are on the Hallelujah Diet. So far I have lost thirteen pounds, and I feel better than I have in years. We are not totally 100% on the diet but are headed in that direction. Two of our sons are on the diet and are doing very well sticking with it. They are fourteen and fifteen years old. My wife Mary says the best thing about the diet is getting up in the morning and feeling good instead of feeling tired. Thanks for the encouragement everyday, it sure has helped us a lot.

Time for today's recipe from Rhonda Malkmus:

• • •

Celery Chowder

    4 stalks of celery
    4 green onions
    1/2 bell pepper
    1 cup carrot juice
    1 Tbsp. minced parsley
    1 small zucchini
    1 Tbsp. parsley
    1 clove of garlic
    1/2 cup celery juice
    Bragg Liquid Aminos to taste (optional)

Dice all vegetables, mince garlic. Blend half of the vegetables with the juices, add the remaining vegetables, minced parsley and Bragg Liquid Aminos to taste.

• • •

I'll see you tomorrow with our Day Twelve Newsletter.

Day Twelve of Our Twenty–One Days to Health the Hallelujah Diet Way

"Let the words of my mouth, and the MEDITATION of my heart, be acceptable in thy sight, O Lord, my strength, and my redeemer" (Psalm 19:14).

Good morning, fellow Hallelujah Health Seeker. Today I want to say a few words about meditation and its relation to building ultimate health.

To begin, let me call on Dr. Malkmus to give us an overview of his thinking on meditation and its place here at Hallelujah Acres.

Dr. Malkmus writes, "The word 'meditation' does not necessarily have a negative connotation. *Webster's Dictionary* defines: 'meditate—to focus one's thoughts on; reflect on or ponder over; to plan or project in the mind; to engage in contemplation…' While the word 'meditation' is defined as 'the act or process of meditating; a discourse intended to express its author's reflections or to guide others in contemplation."

Dr. Malkmus continues: "The Bible often speaks about the importance of spending time in this frame of mind:

I Samuel 9:27: "…but stand thou still a while, that I may show thee the word of God."

Job 37:14: "…Stand still, and consider the wondrous works of God."

Psalm 37:14: "commune with your own heart upon your bed, and be still."

Psalm 46:10: "be still, and know that I am God…"

Philippians 4:8: "Finally, brethren, whatsoever things are true, whatsoever things are honest, whatsoever things are just, whatsoever things are pure, whatsoever things are lovely, whatsoever things are of good report: if there be any virtue, and if there be any praise, think on these things."

Dr. Malkmus concludes, "The Bible clearly shows that there is a time for us to talk to God through the means of prayer. And there should also be a time when we allow God to talk to us through His word, the Bible. And there should also be times when we allow ourselves to communicate with ourselves and reflect on who we are and where we are going. In addition, there should be times when we just are plain still and turn off the world as well as our minds. Meditation and stillness can have great physical and psychological healing properties."

Today I'd like to share with you what I've learned about being still and turning off our minds through meditation or complete relaxation.

If you're like me, you feel terrible for the millions of people in our rush–rush society who are plagued by non–physical health problems, many of which are brought on by stress.

How many friends and relatives do you know who have to take pills every day to deal with depression, insomnia, mood swings, and other mental health challenges?

Did you know that Prozac and Valium and other psychoactive mood drugs are dispensed literally hundreds of thousands of times a day by physicians across our nation to millions of our brothers and sisters who can no longer deal with the stresses of modern life on their own?

Well, the Hallelujah Diet often dramatically improves or heals non–physical problems as beautifully as it heals physical ones.

One of the techniques we recommend for our lifestyle program to help reduce the stress of modern life involves a period of deep relaxation every day, what we call a meditation period.

Research studies have found that twenty minutes of meditation can relax a person better than pills and as well as exercise, in some cases.

Dr. Dean Ornish, one of the great medical doctors of our time who has done so much to bring nutritional and lifestyle healing to America, has daily meditation as one of the keystones of his health program for heart patients. So does Dr. John McDougall, another medical doctor who uses nutrition to heal chronic illness.

And we recommend the same thing here at Hallelujah Acres.

Okay, enough background. You probably want to know how to achieve this state of relaxation that benefits the body almost as much as a long, deep sleep.

Well, it's easy and difficult at the same time.

Easy because you can learn the technique in a matter of seconds and difficult because most of us are so wired and hyperkinetic that it takes days or sometimes even weeks of practicing meditation before we slow down enough to enjoy it.

I'd advise anyone starting meditation to approach it from the same practical angle as you're approaching the 21–day contract. Make a commitment to yourself to meditate for at least five minutes every single day for 21 straight days. And if you miss a day, then you start over again.

What's the simplest way to meditate?

It's called breath counting and you do it like this.

First, find a comfortable spot in a quiet place in your home.

With two teenage boys who enjoy joking around, a wife who loves to talk, and a husband who will yap your ear off most of the time, it's not easy to find quiet in the house where we live unless you sneak into the attic above the garage.

Consequently, I meditate just before I go to bed, when things finally start to quiet down around our place.

Find a comfortable place to sit and be sure to have your spine straight. If you sit in a chair, place your feet flat on the floor.

Lying down to meditate is a no–no since most people will enter the sleep state instead of the relaxation state.

Once you're sitting comfortably, either on a cushion, folded blanket, or straight–backed chair, check to see that your spine is straight. If you tuck your chin in and push your chest out a bit, you'll achieve the proper position.

Oh yes, be sure to have a watch or clock within sight so you can keep track of time. I have a $25 jogging watch that I use. When I sit down to meditate, I push the alarm button, which I have set for 30 minutes. When the watch starts beeping, I know it's time to stop.

You will probably do best to start with a five–minute period of meditation and work up to longer periods as you feel comfortable. I started with two–minute periods back in 1980 and gradually worked up to 30 minutes at a time.

Most folks just plain can't sit without moving for much more than five minutes when they first start.

That's how programmed we are to move, move, move and rush, rush, rush.

Whoa, slow down and haul in the reins. Relax and be still for five minutes a day. Doing so makes a tremendous difference in overall health and peace of mind.

So be patient with yourself and work up to 15–20 minutes per day of meditation.

And don't despair if you have a tough time of it at first. Like the diet and like exercise, meditation gets easier with practice and as you see the good it can do for you. I had a terrible time at first because I had such an active mind and such a wired metabolism (and remember I started meditating when I was still living on Dominos pizza and Big Macs and cherry Danish). But I'm a stubborn guy and I was convinced meditating would help me deal with stress, and it did. Eventually. But I had to really force myself to do it the first couple of weeks, believe me. After I started realizing the benefits, however, it got easier and easier, and that'll be true for you too. I hope.

Okay, here we go.

Once you're in a comfortable, straight–backed position, with your hands folded in your lap or resting lightly on your knees, take a long deep breath and slowly let it out. Do this a second time. Do it a third time.

Be very conscious of your body.

You will feel yourself relaxing as you take these deep breaths.

Remarkably, and sadly, most of us are so busy during our lives that we never become aware of our bodies and the constant signals they send us.

But it's true. Our bodies are communicating with us every second of our lives, and it's only when we're silent and still enough to listen that we actually begin to learn what our bodies need and want.

Now that you're settled in, to begin meditating, close your eyes and breathe normally through your nose.

Your breathing will naturally slow down as the meditation progresses.

Silently, but with your fullest attention, count your breaths, like this:

As you inhale, think, "One."

As you exhale, think, "Two.

As you inhale, think, "Three."

As you exhale, think, "Four."

Continue breathing and counting until you get to ten and then start over again with one.

If you lose track of the count, you don't have to stop and visit a psychiatrist. It's normal to lose track, especially when you start. I've been meditating like this for eighteen years as of this week, and I still lose track of the count sometimes.

If you lose your place, just go back to the last number you remember and begin again.

Especially when you're a novice, other thoughts will race through your mind. When this happens, just return your attention to your breathing and counting.

We all get distracted when relaxing like this. When the distractions come, please shoo them away courteously, without guilt or irritation.

One cool thing about distractions is that if you try to control them, this in itself becomes another distraction. So just count your breaths. Nothing else.

Although you want to remain as still as possible, I won't hand out demerits if you yawn or shift positions or scratch or something. But do try to be as still as possible. From the way I jabber on all the time, you may find it hard to believe, but I can sit for 30 minutes without moving a single muscle or even a hair. I mean, seriously, after all these years of practice, I can be still as stone when I meditate.

Keep your back, neck, and head straight. Stay awake but also stay relaxed. Enjoy what you're doing.

If you haven't set an alarm clock or timer or something, when you think of time, glance at your watch or clock.

When you've had enough or when the time you've set aside for meditating is over, slowly return to your normal thoughts and activities. Because you'll be more relaxed than you've been in a long time (at least after you get the hang of meditating), please wait a few moments before you get up and go back to your regular life. This is one reason I like to meditate just before bed.

I get up from my cushion and crawl under the covers, and I'm literally asleep in minutes—if it takes that long.

And that's all there is to the breath counting meditation.

There are a zillion different meditation methods, and I've experimented with a lot of them, but I always come back to breath counting because it allows me to focus on being still better than any of the other techniques I've tried.

Time for today's recipes from Rhonda's book, *Recipes for Life... from God's Garden:*

• • •

Carrot–Vegetable Juice

Clean and prepare 3/4 lb. of carrots, 1/2 beet with tops, 1 stalk of celery cut into half–inch pieces, along with a handful of your favorite greens like spinach, kale, lettuce, or cabbage. Process in your juicer and enjoy. Serving size is 8 ounces.

• • •

Carrot Soup

2 cups of carrots
1/4 cup red pepper
1/2 cup celery
1/4 tsp. paprika
1/4 cup red onion
1/4 cup broccoli florets
1 cup fresh carrot juice
1/2 tsp. thyme
Bragg Liquid Aminos to taste (optional)

Clean and grate carrots, and finely chop onion, red pepper, broccoli and celery. Mix together. Add carrot juice, Braggs and seasonings. Stir to blend.

And here are a couple of great letters to finish off Day Twelve:

• • •

Chet:

I just wanted to write a note and express my excitement with how this 21–day contract is going. My husband Scott and I both are following the Hallelujah Diet with you. We are very pleased with how everything is going. Many of the things we have experienced have already been expressed by others. But I just couldn't help but share what has been going on here. My husband and I both have been amazed with the energy we have, the lack of cravings (I was a sugar addict), and the lack of hunger. This is the most balanced I have felt since I can remember.

• • •

Dear Chet:

I keep reading about all the wonderful things that are happening for everyone— and just keep saying "Ditto" for myself. I am enjoying this whole process so much—no feeling of deprivation at all. I've lost fifteen pounds and feel wonderful. Loads of energy! Arthritis and sinus problems are improving daily, and I wake up every morning ready to tackle the day. I could go on and on, but it's evident you hear this level of excitement every time you read an e-mail.

I'm so thankful to my friend Dorine for aiming me in this direction. My approaching 58th birthday isn't even daunting now!

• • •

And that takes care of Day Twelve.
See you tomorrow.

Day Thirteen of Our Twenty–One Days to Health the Hallelujah Diet Way

I hope you feel as good as I do.

I'm going to be brief today because I've been working pretty long hours the past two weeks and am ready to practice what I preach in these letters about taking it easy on occasion.

So if this Saturday's newsletter seems dashed off to you, it's because I dashed it off since I wanted to dash off and have some fun with my wife and kids. It's a bit after five a.m. as I write these words, and the last weather forecast I heard said North Carolina was going to actually see the sun today, so guess who's gonna go out hiking in it?

Do YOU have plans to get outside today to get some sun? If it's the dead of winter, you're allowed and encouraged to stay in and stay warm. But if you're not iced or frozen in, why not join me today and tomorrow in at least getting some brisk walking outside in the sun?

Okay, today's tip.

On many Friday nights, my wife and kids start hollering at me, "Dad, Dad, it's Friday night. Let's go out to eat."

I usually start groaning and mumbling things about over–cooked, Standard American Diet garbage, and how I'd much rather stay home and prepare a live dinner than sit in some morgue of a restaurant and watch other people stuff their faces with so–called foods that looked like they just came out of a crematorium.

"Don't be so weird, Dad. We'll go to the place where you can get a salad bar," one of my sons suggests.

I groan some more and roll my eyes, thinking, "Gimme a break—no salad bar can touch the salad I can make at home."

Then I think about how much money I could save if we ate at home instead of going out, and the groan becomes audible.

"He's thinking about the money now," Number Two son remarks casually.

"Come on, Pop, you haven't taken us out for a long time. You need some social life," Number One son advises.

I start to tell them about the last time I dined with the Vanderbilts but then relent.

He's right. I haven't taken them out in quite a while.

So we pack into the car and drive to Ryan's Steak House. In the parking lot, I bang my head on the steering wheel a few times.

"What's the matter?" my wife asks.

"I can't take it, I can't go in there and watch everyone loading their plates with meat and greasy garbage."

"Let's go to the Chinese restaurant in the mall," Number Two son suggests, "we haven't been there before."

He's right.

I relent and we drive to the mall to the Chinese buffet dinner.

I groan when we get there because the sign outside the door says, "Buffet: $7.50 each. Drinks included."

"Seven–fifty each!" I shout. "Seven–fifty! Do you know how many Chinese peasants we could feed for seven–fifty? Heck, you could buy egg rolls for the entire Seventh Fleet for seven–fifty!"

The boys remind me that we're not in China, and my wife rolls her eyes and twirls an index finger by her ear at a passing couple who stopped to stare and listen to my tirade.

I finally settle down, and we enter the restaurant and have a very nice dinner in quiet, unpacked surroundings. Unlike Ryans, which, on a Friday night, always reminds me of a feedlot full of braying cattle.

Okay, okay, so I'm not going to get off a quick tip today—so I'm having too much fun writing this one to dash it off in a hurry!

So sue me.

Anyway, I want to share a few thoughts on how to successfully go out with other people and still remain true to your health program. It's not always easy to go to a restaurant and stick with healthful foods because most restaurants don't have any healthful foods.

Shoot, my wife and I went to a place in downtown Shelby a month or so ago, and they didn't have a single item on the menu that didn't have meat.

I still remember my conversation with the waitress...

"I'd like the taco salad but without meat."

"You don't want any meat?"

"Right. Taco salad with no meat. Just beans. Do the beans contain lard?"

She looks at me. "Whatya say?"

"Lard. Do the refried beans in the taco salad contain lard? You know, animal fat, like in meat."

"What kinda meat you want, chicken or beef?"

"No, no, I don't want any meat. I want to know if the beans contain lard."

"Lord knows," she says, looking at my wife, wondering how such an obviously intelligent and attractive woman could be married to this idiot.

"Okay, just bring the taco salad with no meat and no beans."

"You sure you don't want meat?"

"I'm sure. And I don't want any cheese either."

She looks up from her pad. "No cheese? No meat? How you gonna get your protein?"

I explain to her that protein exists in just about every food and that I drink quarts of carrot juice every day and get some of the most assimilable protein around by doing so.

"We don't have carrot juice," she explains. "You want a Pepsi?"

I tell her I don't drink soft drinks, that I only drink freshly extracted fruit and vegetable juices and distilled water.

"Okay," she says, squirming at this point because she's been told mental illness is sometimes catching. "You want a taco salad with no meat and no cheese, right?"

"And no onions and no olives either," I add. "Just fill the shell with lots of lettuce and as many raw vegetables as the chef has available."

"We don't have a chef here, he's a cook," she explains patiently, "and I don't think we have any raw vegetables either. We get 'em in these big frozen boxes—you know, it says Honduras on the side—you don't want no frozen vegetables, do you?"

At this point, my shin's about to break in half because of the number of times my wife has kicked it under the table.

I look at my beloved of almost 26 years and capitulate.

"Okay, a taco salad shell with lots of lettuce would be great," I say, doing my best to smile at the waitress.

"You have to pay the same price," she explains, her look of concern deepening. "You can still have the meat and cheese—it'll taste a lot better. And you get free refills on that Pepsi!"

"He'll be fine," my wife says, patting the back of my hand, smiling sweetly at the waitress, taking over with her usual good grace and courtesy and extricating me from potentially ending up in either handcuffs or a straitjacket.

Well, I digress.

Anyway, we ate at the Chinese joint last night, and we had a great time.

And you can have a great time at restaurants also—as long as you maintain your sense of humor.

For me, that's one of the keys to dining out while trying to live healthfully.

Another key is to avoid the non–foods that tempt you.

I used to hate to go out because I was always so tempted by so many poor food choices.

But, you know, the past two weeks while I've been on the contract, we've eaten out both Friday nights and I haven't had any problems at all. I had a big salad the night we ate at the steak house, and last night when we went Chinese, I had a big salad followed by vegetable lo–mein. (Remember if you go to a Chinese restaurant, however, to request food with no MSG and those who are soy sensitive need to be careful too.)

And when I got home I had a couple pieces of whole wheat toast with some grapeseed oil on top—yum.

How do you avoid temptations while eating out?

You know, when I started writing this piece I thought I was going to provide all kinds of good "how to" answers to that question.

Things like—stay at the salad bar and don't venture near the buffet.

Ask the waitress to have the chef steam you some vegetables and then put them on a plate of rice.

Order a baked potato or two and eat them with lentil and sunflower sprouts that you brought from home.

And suggestions like that.

But it dawns on me right now that the question really boils down to a simple matter of realizing that poor food choices make you feel bad.

I mean, I would have felt sluggish and dull this morning if I'd eaten most of the stuff at the Chinese buffet. And I remember thinking to myself last night at the restaurant that I didn't want to be sluggish and dull on Saturday.

So I ate the right things, woke up feeling great at five a.m., and here I am a couple hours later almost done with the Day Thirteen letter.

You see, making good choices and living correctly has wonderful pay–offs. It's better than having the Publisher's Clearinghouse Team show up at your door with a check for $10,000,000.

Well, maybe not that good.

But, when you're dining out, before you order the Peiking Duck with orange sauce and braised baby back ribs, just think of how you'll feel the morning after you have the "treat."

My friend, that's one of the glorious thing about having this diet and lifestyle knowledge—once you know how to live and eat healthfully and once you do it for a few weeks, you're touched for life.

Sure you can always go back and eat the Standard American Diet if you want to, and if you want to have chronic ailments in your old age—but you can also stick with the Hallelujah Diet and feel great all the time.

And isn't that an easy choice?

So the next time you eat out—make good choices and feel like a stick of dynamite with a burning fuse the next day.

How about some letters?

• • •

Hey, Chet:

I've had people say, "It's too expensive to eat all those vegetables and fruits."

Once a month I have to do the shopping for my company, stocking up on all the candy and pop they want for their snacks.

I shopped at the wholesale store last night with two carts—one for my FOOD and one for the company's dead stuff, filling both to major capacity.

ALIVE CART total came to $36.70 for 10 items

DEAD CART total came to $99.32 for 18 items

• • •

Dear Chet:

I did put in a contract for 21 days, but I intend to do it for the next 21 years and more. It has helped us in so many ways: more energy, no more sinus headaches, arthritis a lot better, no morning stiffness, no pills since the end of January 1997, stiff knees no longer stiff and so many more things. No way would I ever want to go back to the old way of eating and gain back all the consequences. I tell people if you want to lose some weight you can do so by going on some other diet and still eat your "favorite foods," but you will not lose all the physical problems. I went on weight watchers and I lost the weight but I didn't lose those other problems.

Your taste buds really do change, don't they? My husband is eating food that he never thought he would eat and he is LIKING it. We love our fruit salads for lunch!

• • •

Are you ready for today's recipe from Rhonda Malkmus? Well, ready or not, here's how Rhonda prepares Peiking Duck! Of course, I'm kidding. Instead of munching down on grilled animal skin that's been baked for 24 hours, why don't you instead have something alive and delicious, something like...

• • •

Raw Sweet Corn Salad

1 large ear of raw sweet corn
1/2 red bell pepper, chopped
1 large ripe tomato, diced
3 Tbsp. parsley, minced
1 celery stalk, diced
1/4 cup sweet red onion, chopped

Wash all vegetables, remove kernels of corn from cob, dice tomato, dice celery, chop red pepper and onion, and mince the parsley. Combine in a bowl, cover and set in refrigerator while preparing avocado dressing (see page 68).

Hint: Raw corn on or off the cob is delicious. Simply clean, wash and enjoy.

• • •

Okay, my friend, that's it for today. Please have a great day and enjoy the people around you and be loving to them. Feeding the heart this way is just as important as feeding the body.

See you tomorrow, when we celebrate our second week of success on the Hallelujah Diet.

Day Fourteen of Our Twenty–One Days to Health the Hallelujah Diet Way

Good morning, fellow Hallelujah Health Seeker.

Give yourself a big pat on the back today because we're now two thirds of the way through the 21–day contract.

It's almost 6:30 a.m. here in the den of my home in Shelby, North Carolina, and I'm about to have a big ole tablespoon of Barleygreen for breakfast.

Just pop that powder in the ole mouth and swirl around until it's good and liquid and then, gulp, down the hatch.

Yummy!

What, what's that?

Did I hear the word "Yuck" out there from someone?

Surely not.

Barleygreen tastes great right out of the jar.

Okay, okay, maybe it tastes great right out of the jar after you acquire a taste for it—but do remember that's the best way to have it. Second best is to stir into a couple of ounces of distilled water.

Please be sure you're NOT drinking it with any kind of citrus juice or with cranberry juice because the acidic nature of these choices will neutralize much of the alkaline goodness of the Barleygreen.

Today I'm going to use our Day Fourteen Newsletter to share some food ideas with you.

Let's turn our attention to several of Rhonda Malkmus' great recipes, shall we?

Avocado Salad Pita Pocket

Pita pockets are wonderful! One of my favorites is this live, all–raw recipe: Spread Pita bread with mashed avocado and stuffed with your favorite fresh veggies—diced tomatoes, sprouts, lettuce, cucumber, shredded carrots, etc. Add favorite salad dressing.

• • •

Lentil Almond Loaf

The Loaf

    2 cups soaked lentils
    1/2 cup parsley
    1/2 cup celery
    1/2 cup red onion
    1/2 cup carrots
    1/2 avocado (optional)
    1 1/2 Tbsp. Bragg Liquid Aminos
    1/2 cup tomato (optional)

1 tsp. garlic
1/2 tsp. herb seasoning
1/2 Tbsp. lemon juice
1/4 cup oat bran
The Binder
2 Tbsp. agar agar
1/3 cup distilled water
The Garnish
1/2 cup slivered almonds
cherry tomatoes
sliced cucumbers

Place lentils in enough distilled water to cover and soak overnight. Drain. Mince garlic, shred carrots, dice tomato, chop parsley, celery and onion. Place lentils and other ingredients in a food processor and blend until thoroughly mixed, leave in processor.

Place the agar agar flakes in a small pan with distilled water, mix well and bring to a boil for 1 minute, remove from heat. Allow to cool slightly. Turn on food processor and pour agar agar over the lentil mixture, mix well.

Spoon the lentil mixture onto a lightly oiled sheet of wax paper and roll into a log. Tuck in the ends and place in a bread pan. Refrigerate at least one hour. Unwrap loaf and roll in slivered almonds until covered. Place loaf on a bed of greens with cherry tomatoes and/or sliced cucumbers as garnish.

• • •

Sprouted Grain Crisps

Raw crackers can be made by using any grain, such as wheat, rye, oats, rice, millet or barley. An example would be:

1/4—1/2 cup rye
1 1/2—1 3/4 cup wheat berries
3 cups distilled water

Put the above ingredients in a bowl and soak overnight (about 12 hours). Drain the water, reserving the soak water for use later (do not refrigerate). Place drained grains on a paper towel placed in the bottom of a bowl, cover with a towel and allow to sprout for about 12 hours. When the sprouts are ready, assemble:

1 cup sprouted grains
1 cup soak water
1 Tbsp. dehydrated onions
1 tsp. dill weed
1 tsp. caraway seeds
1 Tbsp. Bragg Liquid Aminos (optional)

Put the above ingredients in a blender and blend until a creamy consistency is reached. Then pour a thin layer onto a plastic dehydrator tray and dehydrate until crisp. (Make sure all moisture has dried before removing from dehydrator tray.) Enjoy with your favorite salad, use as a snack food, or you can make delicious mini–sandwiches by spreading with ripe avocado topped with a dehydrated tomato. These grain–crisps will keep for months in a tightly–sealed container. Note: You can vary the flavor by changing grains, herbs and seasonings. A sweet grain–crisp can be made by adding a ripe banana and pitted dates or raisins to the grains while in the blender. The sweet grain–crisps take longer to dehydrate.

• • •

Sweet Almond Milk

    1 cup almonds, soaked
    6 cups distilled water
    3–4 dates, pitted

Soak almonds overnight and rinse. Blend half the almonds, half the dates and 3 cups of the distilled water. Repeat with remaining ingredients. Pour through a fine strainer to remove the pulp. If being used for an infant, strain through cheese cloth also. Serve at room temperature. Refrigerate any remaining portion. (For plain almond milk, just leave out the dates.)

• • •

Creamy Banana Milk

    1 qt. distilled water
    1/2—1 cup sunflower seeds, soaked overnight
    1/2 ripe banana
    3 Tbsp raisins or 4—5 dates

Place all ingredients in blender and blend for 2 minutes. For a thicker milk, add more banana.

• • •

Okay, my friend, that's it for Day Fourteen.

See you tomorrow, when we start our third and final week of success on our 21–day contract.

Day Fifteen of Our Twenty–One Days to Health the Hallelujah Diet Way

TGIM, everybody.

In case you don't recognize the acronym, it stands for "Thank God It's Monday."

Say what?

Yep, and I know this may sound a little odd, but whereas I used to love the common phrase "Thank God It's Friday," these days one of the mottoes I live by is "Thank God It's Monday."

You see, this phrase summarizes something that I suspected for the first four–plus years of my personal health building but didn't know for sure until June of 1997 when I started working with Dr. Malkmus.

Having work you enjoy may be as important as diet and exercise in building superior health.

I've been thinking about this quite a bit since the middle of 1997, and I'm firmly convinced of its truth, at least in my own case, because my physical, mental, and emotional health have all improved significantly since my work has also become my play.

For the first 25 years of my working life, I taught English in a variety of college prep schools: three in Louisiana and one in Central Florida. I enjoyed working with teenagers, and I loved literature and writing, and I don't have a lot of complaints about those years. I felt as though I was earning an honest living for my family while even doing some good for a few individuals once in a while.

But even though I enjoyed my teaching jobs most of the time, there were a couple of bad years at schools where things weren't quite right; and even at the good schools, there were days when I had to force myself out of bed to go to work.

And during those years I often got what I called "the Sunday blues," a feeling of depression that started around noon on Sunday and just got worse as time for work the next day rolled around. Of course these blues weren't helped by my diet of junk food, soft drinks, and more junk food.

These periods of melancholy improved dramatically when I made my diet and lifestyle changes in 1993, but they didn't go away entirely until June of 1997 when I stopped teaching and started working with Dr. Malkmus.

You see, it was then that my work and my play were no longer separated.

I was finally doing what in my heart I'd wanted to do my entire life, and that was to earn my living by writing.

You know, even on a healthy diet, before I started working with Dr. Malkmus, I occasionally woke up on Monday mornings with a headache or an unsettled stomach or some mysterious feeling of malaise. I'd usually ignore those feelings and pull myself out of bed and go to school, but on other occasions, at least before I started the Hallelujah Diet in June of 1996, I'd call in sick and then spend the day in the sack—and that would sometimes extend over to Tuesday as well.

But these instances are now a thing of the past.

These days I don't get up to go to work—instead I get up to do precisely what I want to do with my life: write about the Hallelujah Diet and lifestyle program and share how most folks can use it to improve their lives.

The gratification and happiness that comes from this work I can hardly express, but I do know I'm finally living the truth of what my father told me when I was growing up: "Find work you love. You'll be miserable in your heart until you do."

Now, please don't think I'm telling you to turn in your resignation if you don't love your job.

I'm not.

I recognize the realities of earning a living in this world, and I also fully understand that it's rarely easy or practical to quit one's job and start over again.

At the same time, if you're not happy with your job, I encourage you to begin to explore options that may allow you somewhere down the line to do as I've done—to make your work your play.

It took me almost five years to transition from teaching school to working with Dr. Malkmus, but once I found my life work of writing about health (and it took me until age 44 to do that) I set a goal for myself at the beginning of those five years to be supporting my family as a writer by the end of ten years.

Thanks to Dr. Malkmus, I reached that goal five years sooner than I had planned.

And you can do the same thing. It's tough, but it's doable if you set a goal and then do whatever's necessary to reach that goal.

So, if you're currently in a job you have to drag yourself out of bed to go to, please start thinking about alternatives. Sit down and figure out where you want to be in five years and what you want to be doing and then start planning your escape route.

Will your health deteriorate if you don't do this?

Yes, to an extent it will.

There are studies galore that prove health is affected by frame of mind, and if you're depressed or blue several hours out of the day, five days a week, it just makes sense that you're not going to experience the kind of happy, vibrant health that explodes you out of the sack in the morning so you can dash off to work and put in however many hours it takes to get the project(s) done that you eagerly planned to do that day.

So, please, my friend, do what you can to make your work your play.

Time to share a few more inspiring letters:

• • •

I started this diet in September but continued to eat chicken, some white flour and some sweets as well as cooked food. What a difference these past two weeks have been for me! For the past several years I have had a host of symptoms... pains... aches... weakness... visual disturbances... fatigue, etc. They have slowly disappeared yet I always had the weakness in my legs which has made me shy away from anything athletic. Yesterday my husband took me snowshoeing for about 1 1/2 hours and it wasn't even a struggle. I could have gone another hour. I am just so amazed at what a difference a raw diet, minus the sugar, meat and white flour makes in one's health.

I've also found my healing to come in increments. I'll get better in some areas and it will remain so with no more changes for quite a while. Then all of a sudden another symptom seems to diminish. It's very gradual yet definite. My husband asked me if I was getting sick of salads yet, but I really look forward to making and eating them now because I see it as another step in healing each time. You REALLY have something to look forward to in this diet! (What the next day brings you as you continue to apply the principles!)

I feel the most important principle in the success of this diet (for me) is the daily support and input. It really is so helpful knowing there are so many other people doing the same thing you are doing and getting great results. Thanks again for helping us achieve optimum health!

• • •

Chet:

I appreciated your comments about the meditation times. I'd like to share some of the ways I use prayer and meditation. In the early morning after I take my Barleygreen, I spend a few minutes reading the Bible (I'm reading through the Bible. I don't read enough chapters daily to read it in a year, but I eventually get through it). I spend a few minutes meditating on these passages and praying for concerns.

One of the other things I've done in this area is write about 30 or 35 Bible verses related to health and healing on note cards (one per note card) and when I go walking, I flip through these as I walk, and I pray or meditate on these verses. I breathe deeply and regularly as I walk and I consider this prayer/meditation time. Sometimes, I just repeat a favorite verse or Bible phrase over and over as I walk (such as, The Lord is my Shepherd, I shall not want).

Sometimes, later in the day, I sit quietly, read a Psalm, and meditate on that Psalm—quieting myself, breathing deeply and regularly. This is great as a Stress Break. I've memorized several Psalms this way.

I'd also like to share a tip for those of us who really miss our morning cereal. I chop up an apple and/or a pear into a bowl, a few banana slices, add some raisins or chopped dates, a few (very few) chopped almonds, add a little orange juice or rice or soy milk and Voila! you have morning fruit "cereal." It works for me!

• • •

How about a recipe or two? Let's begin with Rhonda Malkmus' tasty…

• • •

Avocado Dressing

    1 ripe avocado
    1 lemon, juiced
Mash the avocado until smooth, add the lemon juice until a creamy consistency is obtained.

    To Serve: Place leaf lettuce on a plate, spread with avocado mixture, top with raw sweet corn salad.

• • •

Raw Corn Chowder

    4 cups fresh corn kernels
    1 cup zucchini
    2 medium tomatoes
    4 green onions
    1/2 bell pepper
    1 stalk of celery
    1 cup fresh carrot juice
    1/4 tsp. thyme
    1/2 tsp. basil
    1 Tbsp. Bragg Liquid Aminos (optional)
Cut the corn from the cob and scrape the cob to obtain what is left behind. Peel and chop tomatoes into small pieces, grate zucchini, chop onions and pepper, and dice celery. Place 1/3 of the ingredients in a blender, blend until creamy, and add to chowder. Fold in remaining ingredients and serve at room temperature.

• • •

Okey dokey, that does it for Day Fifteen. Tomorrow I'm going to turn our attention to something I call "energy sinks." I want to provide a few tips on how to deal with the annoying situations and relationships that turn up in life, the moments of frustration that can gobble good moods and energy in a split second. Until then, enjoy this beautiful day and the rest of this great week.

Day Sixteen of Our Twenty–One Days to Health the Hallelujah Diet Way

Today's topic: energy sinks.

You know—that new kitchen appliance advertised on the infomercials?

The one you can buy with the tiny atomic motor that'll wash your dishes while also disposing of carrot pulp—the one that drains dish water like a Texas tornado.

You know.

Energy sinks.

Hahaha.

Okay, okay, I know, call in the men in white coats. Let's get a tailor working on a jacket for Chet—one of those nice white jackets in the stiff material with the sleeves that tie so neatly behind the back.

I'll stop.

You see, I just woke up feeling so good this morning that I've been dying to crack a joke for two hours. And nobody's here at work yet to share a laugh with, so I let you have it.

For the rest of this letter, I'll try to keep the stretching confined to the body and not to the jokes.

Seriously, though, I do want to spend a few minutes writing about energy sinks.

When I use the term "energy sinks," I'm referring to those moments or relationships or incidents that occur all the time in life that will gobble up your energy quicker than an elephant falling into an Olympic–sized pool of quicksand.

I can write about this topic with some authority because I've had a problem dealing with energy sinks for most of my life. I still have the problem, though I'm getting better about it with time and constant conscious effort to improve.

Energy sinks occur most often in people who try to please everyone all the time. Statistically, if, like me, you are the first child in a family, you have a better chance of being affected by energy sinks than your siblings do.

Why?

Because the eldest child in a family usually tries to please everyone in the family as much of the time as possible. And this desire to please carries over into adulthood.

If you're trying to please everyone all the time, you've put yourself in a no–win situation. Because no matter how hard you try and how hard you work and how good of a person you try to be, you're just plain not going to please everyone all the time.

And if you persist in trying to please everyone all the time, you've opened yourself to constant energy sinks.

An energy sink, then, represents a position where you are going to squander some of the energy you have for the day on a situation which doesn't deserve the energy you're giving it.

Example of one of my typical energy sinks: I get an e–mail from a meat eater who criticizes my approach to writing one of the daily health tips. This person insists I am wrong and potentially harming other people. He gives no recognition to my experience or to my years of study in the alternative health field or to my desire to share the health message with anyone who will listen.

In no uncertain terms, he flat out informs me that folks must eat meat three times a day to get their protein. He knows this to be a fact, and he knows I am wrong in what I'm teaching.

If I don't publicly retract what I'm saying immediately, he threatens to tell everyone he knows that my writing is dangerous and that they shouldn't read it.

Now, my friends, this little piece of e–mail represents a classic energy sink.

(And one of the keys to dealing with energy sinks is to recognize them when they arrive and not after they've drained you and left you tense and half ex-hausted.)

A few years ago, I would have dropped everything I was doing and would have spent hours trying to explain my point of view. You see, in those days, I not only still wanted to please everyone, but I also still thought it was possible to please everyone if I just made myself clear enough.

I hadn't yet learned that some people aren't as open–minded as others, and that some folks are so entrenched in their points of view that no matter what you say to them you can't move them off the hard rock they're standing on.

Of course, the letter I spent hours writing might or might not be read with any degree of attention, but you can be sure a response would be forthcoming that would require more thought and more writing, and this might continue for days.

A classic energy sink.

Was anything gained by this dialogue?

No, not really, since both parties had points of view they considered the correct one.

Was anything lost by this dialogue?

Yes, hours and hours of time and energy that would have done more good had both of us involved in the energy sink used that time and energy for some-thing other than to argue our particular point of view.

So these days, when I get an energy sink letter in my e–mail box, I thank the person politely for sharing his or her thoughts, and I then move on about my business, taking care of anywhere from the 60 to 150 or more e–mails that I receive every day of the week.

But do I reject what the energy sink letters say?

Not at all, and this is an important point for learning to deal with energy sinks.

By not engaging in the energy sink, you save valuable time and nerve power; but by ignoring what the person had to say, you may miss a possible opportunity for growth.

So I always read and think carefully about what everyone says to me since one of my goals in life is to improve each day as much as I can, but I don't let aggressive and critical comments, situations, or relationships take away too much of that day's storehouse of energy.

In other words, I learn what I can from each situation, but I don't get bogged down in conflict.

Am I making any sense? Are you following what I'm trying to say?

Another potential energy sink.

If you've been married almost 26 years, as I have, then you know there are absolutely no energy sinks in married or family life.

Right?

Hahahaha, just kidding on that one.

Of course there are energy sinks in a marriage and family life, and if a husband and wife and the children don't learn to recognize them and deal with them, then that marriage and family is doomed from the start, in my opinion.

What if two very stubborn people happen to end up together at the hitching post?

Then they must learn to compromise or else learn to let go of the potential energy sinks.

For example, my wife and I are both stubborn as oak beams in steel–reinforced concrete.

When one of us knows we're right, there's not much give.

Our stubborn natures could have wiped us out many years ago, but we quickly realized that when we run into one of these no–win situations, the best thing to do is to agree to disagree and to then move on to something else.

This way we avoid energy sinks that exhaust so many couples and marriages.

Hey, I'm not a trained psychologist or marriage counselor and what I just wrote may violate all kinds of rules for the marriage road. I dunno. What I do know is that the techniques we've developed over the years for our marriage have kept us together longer than any of our friends in college. Indeed, almost all our friends from those days divorced long ago. So we must be doing something right.

Okay, enough on energy sinks. I do hope you'll give the topic some thought, however, because there's only so much energy available to us each day, and I believe we need to learn to use that energy as constructively and lovingly as possible.

Time for a couple of great letters.

• • •

Dear Chet:

I certainly did not eat very well the month of December. I weighed in at 334 pounds.

I knew I needed to do something and along came your 21 day challenge! My daughter and I took the challenge to change our way of eating to God's way of eating. We have had some hard times but have been encouraged to continue with your newsletters and our results. We have not weighed since beginning the healthy way of eating. I plan on returning to the doctor's office the end of January and I'll weigh then.

My daughter and I have taken our measurements. By the end of two weeks she has lost 4 inches in her waist, two inches in her hips and one inch in her bust. I have lost 4 inches in my hips, 2 inches in my waist, and 2 inches in my bust. We are thankful to you.

We have been walking at least six days out of seven. I started out walking the mile in 33 minutes. No record breaker here! We now have the mile down to 22 minutes. We are working on the 15 min. mile—what a challenge for us but we know that we will make it.

I also know that my temple is getting a renovation! Praise God. I will feel better after fifty than I have ever felt in my life. My daughter is nineteen and now has hope for a healthy future.

• • •

Chet:

This is Day 15 for me. Six more days till the end of the contract and I can eat whatever I want after this! I can hardly wait! I think on Day 22 (the day after the contract ends) I'll just go crazy and stuff myself with all the food I so desire! Maybe I'll start with Barleygreen in the morning, and then (30 min. later) a Granny Smith apple. For lunch I'll probably really do it up with more Barleygreen, a large glass of carrot juice, and then a gigantic salad. For dinner—who knows? Another Barleygreen, possibly a baked potato (plain) and an assortment of steamed vegetables.

What I'm trying to say is I can't even imagine ever eating the SAD way again! I do get a little tempted because I live with three SAD eaters, but it would feel like sin to eat the old way again.

I have lost maybe about eight lbs., but the most noticeable difference has been the inches I've lost. I didn't measure myself before we started—I can tell by how my clothes fit. They're getting loose! (Even though I wasn't too overweight to start with.)

My children tell me that I've been so much "nicer" lately too.

I cringe when I watch my husband and children eat SADly. I know, though, that this new lifestyle is a testimony to them. As time goes on maybe they, too, will have a desire to live and feel better.

• • •

We haven't had a good joke lately, so rather than one of my feeble stretches, let's tickle the ole funny bones with a funny story that came in the mail today:

A seaman met a pirate in a bar, and talk turned to their adventures on the sea. The seaman noted that the pirate had a peg leg, a hook, and an eye patch.

The seaman asked, "So, how did you end up with the peg leg?"

The pirate replied, "We were in a storm at sea, and I was swept overboard into a school of sharks. Just as my men were pulling me out, a shark bit my leg off."

"Wow!" said the seaman. "What about your hook?"

"Well," replied the pirate, "we were boarding an enemy ship and were battling the other sailors with swords. One of the enemy cut my hand off."

"Incredible!" remarked the seaman. "How did you get the eye patch?"

"A seagull dropping fell into my eye," replied the pirate.

"You lost your eye to a seagull dropping?" the sailor asked incredulously.

"Well," said the pirate, "you see, it was my first day with the hook."

• • •

And let's end this day's tip with a wonderful live recipe from Rhonda Malkmus' recipe book:

• • •

Borscht

    1 cup shredded beets
    1 small onion or 2 green onions
    3/4 cup fresh carrot juice
    1 medium tomato
    1 stalk of celery
    1/4 cup fresh beet juice
    1/2 tsp. dill weed
    1/4 head medium cabbage

Shred beets and cabbage and set aside. Peel and chop tomato, chop celery and onion, place in blender with juices, blend until smooth consistency. Mix in dill and pour over shredded beets and cabbage and serve at room temperature.

• • •

We have five days left on the contract, my friend.

Can you believe how fast these three weeks have gone by? I still can't get over it.

Mercy, it's going to be the next century before we know it.

See you tomorrow.

Day Seventeen of Our Twenty–One Days to Health the Hallelujah Diet Way

Whoa.

We've entered the home stretch of our 21–day contract now.

Five more days and we reach the end of the signed commitment.

Unless you fell off the wagon once or twice and had to start over again, but if that happened, then say "Hallelujah!" because you get some extra days on the Hallelujah Diet and even more good health benefits.

Of course, with lifestyle changes of this magnitude, not everything comes up smelling like a rose, and some downsides do accompany the good things.

Today I want to write about one of these downsides, a topic I think you'll find interesting since most of us have to address this issue sooner or later once we have committed ourselves to eating and living properly.

You see, today I'd like to write a few words on *"How to Live Happily on the Hallelujah Diet When Your Family and Friends Think You Need a Psychiatrist."*

Whoa, I think I just heard you say, "That's what I've been dealing with for the past seventeen days."

Well, almost all of us have to deal with this very real and very difficult problem.

I'm not going to recount my own testimony in detail since I've done it before in other places, but, briefly, in 1993, at the age of 44 I found myself unraveling at the seams. At 5'7" tall, I weighed almost 200 lbs and looked like a pear with legs. Arthritis, which runs in my family, started hitting my fingers—bad news for a writer. And I suffered constant pain in my right shoulder, pain that intensified so badly at night that I'd wake up hollering if I rolled over on it. The energy I had enjoyed as a younger man had taken a hike, and I spent too many hours and days feeling blue and sorry for poor old aging me.

So I visited a doctor for the first time in years. The doc offered me pills and injections in the shoulder, both of which I declined. He also told me to get used to physical problems, that I could expect more of them because of my age.

Being a stubborn sort and a self–learner, I rejected his conclusions and decided to look elsewhere for answers. Because my wife had been interested in alternative approaches to health since major cancer surgery in 1990, I decided to read some of her books and to purchase some more at the local health food store.

(I should add that, up to the point where I got interested in taking charge of my own health, I often thought my wife needed a psychiatrist because of the weight she had lost on her crazy vegetarian diet.)

In those days, she followed one diet, and the boys and I ate a lot of pizza and hamburgers if I couldn't stand the thought of yet another big salad followed by something yucky like rice and steamed veggies. I mean, seriously, before I saw the light on health I thought that kind of junk would gag a maggot.

On more occasions than I care to remember I must confess that I treated my wife's ideas about health and diet with nothing but scorn.

Then I read Norman Walker's book on fruit and vegetable juices, and the light bulb literally exploded in my head, and I did the sharpest 180 degree turn you've ever seen a fat man make.

Overnight, in June of 1993, I changed my diet and lifestyle, and by late August of that year, when I started back to the school where I taught high school English, I had lost something like 48 pounds.

Talk about a shadow of his former self.

And I felt great.

I had the energy I'd enjoyed as a teenager. I could go out and run the levees of New Orleans until the cows came home, and my arthritis and shoulder problems had completely healed. Totally gone. I felt like I had a new mind in a new body.

What did I want to do with what I'd learned about health?

Well, of course I wanted to share the knowledge with everybody I knew. Once I realized we didn't have to be sick, I wanted to tell everyone all about it. I wanted everybody on earth to feel the way I felt.

"You look great!" My colleagues at school were happy for me and enthusiastic about my physical changes. "How'd you lose all that weight?"

So I'd tell them they could do what I had done to get the same results—just quit eating meat, dairy products, white flour, salt, and anything with sugar in it. Start exercising in the sunshine every day. Keep the stress level down. And so on.

My friends, their eyes glazed over so fast you could almost hear the eyelids banging together.

Literally within seconds, most of them changed the topic or muttered something about "Gotta get my next period class prepared."

Their response killed me with disappointment and turned me into a nut at the same time.

You see, the more resistant they were to the health message, the more zealous I was in trying to convince them that I had discovered knowledge that could make them not only healthy but supremely energetic and happy.

If I saw one of them eating a candy bar, do you think I could mind my own business about it? Mercy, no. I had to make a comment and then go off on my spiel about the dangers of sugar and chocolate.

If I saw one of them drinking a soft drink, out came my memorized lecture on the horrors of phosphoric acid and caffeine.

If I sat with one of them in the cafeteria and he ate meat, do you think I could manage to keep my mouth shut? Of course not. I felt morally obligated to inform him about the antibiotics and growth hormones and so on in the dead, putrid, rotting flesh he chewed so casually on.

Did I alienate myself from most of my colleagues in a pretty short time?

Well, yes and no.

Yes because they finally made it clear to me that they had heard enough of my health message, and no because they still liked me since I did have a good sense of humor and always had been kind of eccentric and weird anyway.

So I essentially became the school oddball.

Well, before I finally came to my senses and vowed to keep my mouth shut about health unless someone asked me about my approach, I managed to drive a pretty good wedge between myself and my aging and ill parents too. You see, for the past several years, they've been losing their health and dying by inches, and yet they'll have nothing to do with the health knowledge that could liberate them from the diseases and doctors that are killing them.

I found this stubborn refusal to even consider an alternative approach to health the most frustrating thing in my entire life. I love my mom and dad very much, but I can hardly talk to them anymore because all they want to do is tell me about their aches and pains and latest visit to their many doctors and how none of the doctors are helping them and how all the medications are making them sicker, and all I want to do is scream that I can't stand to hear it because it doesn't have to be this way.

This is my big frustration, and I know many of you share it with me, either with parents or with spouse and children or with other family members or even well–meaning friends who think "You're killing yourself. Look how thin you're getting."

Folks, living the Hallelujah Diet and dealing with loved ones and friends I find the hardest part of the whole program.

Seriously, eating five gallons of sandy kelp would be easy in comparison to dealing with loved ones who just plain won't even consider trying a change in diet for a week or two.

And yet we each have to come to terms with this division in thought and lifestyle because if we don't we can literally ruin relationships with family and friends.

I know of marriages that have actually ended because one partner could no longer stand to live with another partner who refused to change his/her diet.

So what do you do when confronted with this difficult problem?

My friends, I'm sorry, but I don't have easy answers for this one.

In my own case, I do the best I can to keep my mouth shut and to love unconditionally those who don't see things my way and who will never make more than token changes. But I foul up with this all the time.

Some days I'm convinced the connection between my mouth and brain has been severed because I'm listening to myself nag a loved one when my brain's asking me, "Why are you doing this? You're not going to help them make better choices by being a jerk about it."

I guess it boils down to being judgmental. When I stop judging others by my standards and accept them and love them for what they are and where they are on the health path, then I do much better than when I mount my high horse and try to trample everyone in sight with the truth.

Yes, I know this tip hasn't come together the way it should. But I just don't know the answers to this question the way I know the answers to some of the others.

I do know Dr. Malkmus spent twenty years in the wilderness, trying to preach the health message to pastors and people who wouldn't listen, and yet he persisted. And because he persisted and didn't give up, thousands now have the health and happiness we wouldn't have had if he had clammed up and never said a word about health to anyone again.

I know Dr. Malkmus' life would have been easier if he had made that choice.

But look what the thousands and thousands on the Hallelujah Diet would have lost had he taken the easy way out.

So I guess we must do what he did—share the health message with anyone who will listen and thus spread it to the world one person at a time.

Even if the people who want to hear "how not to be sick" aren't the loved ones in our families with whom we most want to share it.

Final thoughts.

Try to teach by example rather than by force. Use a fly swatter instead of a baseball bat. Open your heart instead of your mouth.

Be patient because when people see you changing—growing happier, healthier, and more energetic as the days and weeks and months go by—some of them, not all by any means, but some of them will eventually open their minds and hearts and ask you what you're doing.

That's the time to share the knowledge.

But, mercy, it's hard to wait for that moment.

Okay, enough, enough, enough.

Let's finish the day with a great letter, then a quick recipe, and finally a hilarious joke which I trust you'll find as punny as I did.

• • •

Dear Chet:

Although I failed to officially sign up on the 21–day contract, a good friend has been forwarding me the daily newsletters and I am learning great things. Chet, I wanted to give you an update on how my teenager is doing after four months on the Hallelujah Diet. I've told you before he is 17 and wrestles for his high school. Well, his new nickname is "Veggie–Boy" and he is now getting the respect of every coach for several reasons.

First, he doesn't have to struggle to maintain his weight like the guys who lose weight by running miles and miles, wrestle weak, stuff down pizza afterward, and have to lose weight again. This is especially good with all the scares in high school and college wrestling programs with young men dying.

Second, at the end of every practice (which are incredibly tough) Jeremy is the only one left standing or still doing push–ups. Jeremy has never really been a "jock" like most of the guys on the team, but he works hard and never takes the easy way out when running, push–ups, lifting weights, etc. And everyone notices.

Third, we are excited about the fact that Jeremy has received nominations to both the Air Force and Naval Academies—again because he has proved himself a dedicated worker and passed their tough fitness test, passing many of the "jocks" taking the same test. Now we just pray that he will be allowed to continue his commitment to not eating meat and taking Barleygreen wherever he goes next year. Who knows, he might be another Daniel and convince his whole flight to go on the Hallelujah Diet! Imagine if our military academies suddenly became healthier!

BTW, I've now lost 35+ pounds since changing my diet Oct 1, 1997, and this morning I RAN a full mile without stopping or walking! Plus, three months ago I was BEGGING for a hysterectomy and three+ months without chicken and I am as normal as I was 25 years ago…. in fact, BETTER!

• • •

Wasn't that an inspiring testimony?

Time for a recipe. Today I want to share a concoction I put together as part of our dinner last night. It turned out a lot better than I expected, so I offer it for your consideration. Be warned, however, that I tend to prepare meals the way I write—a little of this, a little of that, plug in something here and digress there, and that's how we got—

• • •

Chet's Sweet Potato Delight

> Four baked yams
> Big handful of organic raisins
> Juice of one big navel orange
> Two slices of dehydrated pineapple (fresh would be better)
> Two tablespoons of cherry jam

Bake the yams the day before and refrigerate overnight. Thirty minutes before eating, take the yams out of the frig and smush them in a casserole dish. Add the other ingredients (dice the pineapple) and mix thoroughly. If you like your evening meal hot, slip the covered dish into a 350 degree oven for about thirty minutes. Take the cover off for the last five minutes if you want to brown the top a bit. If you like your evening meal cold, let the covered dish sit on the countertop for thirty minutes so the flavors can blend. Be sure to use a natural, cherry jam that doesn't contain sugar and additives. Serves 3–4 hungry writers.

• • •

And let's finish with a joke that was waiting in my mail this morning.

• • •

Recently a guy in Paris nearly got away with stealing several paintings from the Louvre. However, after planning the crime, getting in and out past security, he was captured only two blocks away when his Econoline ran out of gas. When asked how he could mastermind such a crime and then make such an obvious error, he replied: "I had no Monet to buy Degas to make the Van Gogh."

GROAN…Punny, eh? I told you.

On that note, see you tomorrow for Day Eighteen.

Day Eighteen of Our Twenty–One Days to Health the Hallelujah Diet Way

During the winter, many of us can't bask for twenty minutes in the rays of the sun because ole Sol doesn't come out from behind the clouds for weeks at a time.

Many of us have a hard time getting outside each day for at least twenty minutes of brisk walking or easy jogging. After all, slogging through the snow in Nike Air Chets just plain ain't for everybody.

Breathe clean, fresh air all the time?

Forget about it! Many of us work in buildings that don't even have windows that could be opened by a jack hammer, much less by the muscles of a human being.

Never cheating on the diet? In a world with Godiva Chocolates, Ben & Jerry Garcia's Coffee Toffee Double Dutch Rock–n–Roll Sour Cream Filet Mignon Delight, and Shoney's all–you–can–eat week day breakfast bar for less than a five dollar bill?

Never cheat?

Right. Wink, wink, snicker, snicker.

Having freshly extracted carrot juice three times a day either requires superhuman organization or a part–time employee to make the wonderful stuff.

If you're on your own, to get that juice as often and as optimally as possible, it probably requires getting up an hour early to peel the carrots, juice the juice, take the pulp outside to distribute on the compost heap, turn the compost heap, and then trudge through the snow back to the house to clean up the darn machine.

I bet none of you have even thought about throwing a $600 juicer through the kitchen window instead of taking it apart and cleaning it with those goofy little brushes one more time. Nah, nobody on the contract would ever have that thought.

Well, in the real world of hustle and bustle and ten hour work days and too much stress and not enough rest and relaxation to begin with, not all of us can find the time to juice twice a day the way we should.

Mercy, staying with the Hallelujah Lifestyle does take stamina and determination, doesn't it?

To answer my own question, "Yes it does, and I congratulate you for doing a great job of putting health as a major priority in your life. So pat yourself on the back, raise your hands in the air, and shout Hallelujah!"

But, no question about it, many of the requirements for superior health are tough to consistently squeeze in every day.

Well, to make things a little easier, I have a new requirement for you that you <u>can</u> squeeze in every day, and you can squeeze it in several times a day, and if you don't squeeze in this simple health enhancer every day, you have only yourself to blame.

The requirement?

Why, laughing from deep inside, of course.

My friends, laughter costs nothing, takes no time, requires little effort, and pays off with a jackpot in silver health dollars.

As they so aptly put it in the *Reader's Digest*, "Laughter—the Best Medicine."

I won't go into the "scientific research" that proves laughter has good effects on mental, physical, and emotional health—but the research has been done. If you want to do your own doubleblind study on this, work yourself into a sour mood by watching the nightly news and then go read some of the jokes you'll find at the end of this letter. If you don't feel better after reading the jokes and chuckling aloud a time or two, I'll eat my bicycle seat.

So, on this eighteenth day of our contract, I want to take a break from the serious business of diet and lifestyle changes and health requirements and urge you to have at least one good belly laugh, twenty–five chuckles, and a hundred smiles every day for the rest of your life.

You do *not* have to keep a daily Laugh Journal to document your amusement periods, though the obsessive–compulsive Type–A's like me out there may want to do so just to keep their records up to date.

Friends, other health enhancers on the Hallelujah program take work and discipline, at least until you begin to realize some of the marvelous benefits, but laughter and good humor come naturally.

And if you know some humorless people or if you haven't laughed or smiled since 1973, you can bet a dime to a donut, oops, make that a dime to a radish, that anyone without humor is carrying around a nasty load of toxins. I firmly believe that God designed us with a capacity for laughter for many reasons, not the least of which is to flood the body with hormones and chemicals that help the ole cells yell "Whooooeeeee!"

And if you find your sense of humor increasing as you stick with the Hallelujah lifestyle, don't be at all surprised.

You know you're making serious progress when folks start saying things like "What's going on with you? You're smiling and happy all the time these days."

My dear friend, it's impossible to not laugh and find the world full of fun and joy and love when you've cleaned out your body/temple.

It's just another of God's gifts to us when we live His way instead of the Standard American Diet way.

And what a great gift it is.

For some reason, many people send me jokes and funny lists in e–mail, which I enjoy very much, though I can't imagine why they send them to me since I obviously have no sense of humor.

Anyway, may I share a few of these with you?

If all the salmon caught in Canada in one year were laid end to end across the Sahara Desert, the smell would be absolutely awful.

• • •

From the "Let's Have a Chuckle Poetry Section," we find this submission:

• • •

The Month After Christmas

Twas the month after Christmas, and all through the house
Nothing would fit me, not even a blouse.
The cookies I'd nibbled, the eggnog I'd taste
At the holiday parties had gone to my waist.
When I got on the scales there arose such a number!
When I walked to the store (less a walk than a lumber).
I'd remember the marvelous meals I'd prepared;
The gravies and sauces and beef nicely rared,
The wine and the rum balls, the bread and the cheese
And the way I'd never said, "No thank you, please."
As I dressed myself in my husband's old shirt
And prepared once again to do battle with dirt –
I said to myself, as I only can "You can't spend a winter
disguised as a man!"
So—away with the last of the sour cream dip,
Get rid of the fruit cake, every cracker and chip
Every last bit of food that I like must be banished
Till all the additional ounces have vanished.
I won't have a cookie—not even a lick.
I'll want only to chew on a long celery stick.
I won't have hot biscuits, or corn bread, or pie,
I'll munch on a carrot and quietly cry.
I'm hungry, I'm lonesome, and life is a bore –
But isn't that what January is for?
Unable to giggle, no longer a riot.
Happy New Year to all and to all a good diet!

• • •

And in the humor from real life section, today we have a submission from a fellow contractee, a quick anecdote that cracked me up.

Hanging in the hallway at Jay High School Gym are the basketball team pictures from the past 40 years. A player in the center of the front row in each picture holds a basketball identifying the year—"62–63," "63–64," "64–65," etc. One day I spotted a freshman looking curiously at the photos. Turning to me, he said, "Isn't it strange how the teams always lost by one point?"

Here are a few tips from others on how they share the good news about health with friends and family:

• • •

When I want others to hear about health/diet and I'm not sure how receptive they'll be, I just say I want to tell them about things I'm learning or trying and how it makes sense to me. I'm teaching them as I tell them about my experiences. Since I present it as sharing things I'm excited about instead of telling them they need to hear and learn things, the information is usually well received.

• • •

I really haven't had any problem with my family and friends yet because I immediately tell them I'm on the diet for health reasons, that my body can't handle sugar, white flour meat, etc. It immediately makes them feel less guilty because the problem is more focused on me than them. Then they silently wonder if it would work for them without trying to defend their habits of eating poorly. In the past with other diets my husband and I would get in arguments.

Now, I make my family their SAD meals and they watch every night as I sit down to my huge salad and baked potato. While they are not on the defensive and enjoying their SAD meal, I can slowly sneak in some teaching about the health of raw foods. Someone is always getting sick (but not me) with a cold, strep, joint pain, whatever. Then I teach them how food affects their healing, etc and they really listen.

I love setting the example every night with the fresh veggies and now I make sure they have their salad as part of their meal. (They can handle that much.) Change is long, and slow. Patience is the key. If it takes years for my family to see the light, I am willing to wait as I set the example and they watch my health improve.

Oh… just wanted to mention that when I went snowshoeing the other day… my back "went out." Instead of needing two–three weeks of adjustments, my body only needed one. The healing was so quick that I was totally amazed and thankful.

• • •

And let's finish with a quick recipe from Rhonda's cook book:

• • •

Chinese Vegetables
1 large garlic clove
1 large red onion
1 Tbsp. Bragg Liquid Aminos (optional)
1/3 cup almonds
2 cups celery
1 medium red bell pepper
2 cups Chinese cabbage

Sliver almonds into small slices. Mince garlic, cut celery into thin U–shaped pieces, cut pepper and onion into thin strips and shred Chinese cabbage. On a warmed plate, make a bed of shredded cabbage, top with vegetables and slivered almonds.

Make the following sauce and stir until well blended. Place in a saucepan and heat until thickened, cool slightly, and pour over vegetables.

2 Tbsp. arrow root powder

1/2 cup distilled water

1/4 cup Bragg Liquid Aminos

And that finishes Day Eighteen of our 21–Day Contract.

Day Nineteen of Our Twenty–One Days to Health the Hallelujah Diet Way

Well, this morning I had planned to write about the fun and benefits of dehydrating food, but I've decided to devote this issue instead to two letters that I think you will appreciate and find helpful as you continue with the Hallelujah Diet and lifestyle after the contract commitment ends.

Without further jabbering from me, please find a comfortable chair and read two wonderful letters from Hallelujah Diet enthusiast Kathleen Gabrielle, who took hours out of her busy schedule to share what she's learned with us.

I'll comment in [these brackets] when appropriate.

First, for those of you who want some hints on feeding teenagers:

• • •

What Do You Feed a Veggie–Boy?
by Kathleen Gabrielle

When I tell people I'm a vegetarian they often don't ask questions. But when I mention that my 17–year old son is one, too, they want to know why, how, whose idea it was and many other questions.

The first thing I usually tell people is that my son and I came to the decision to be vegans while in separate locations and listening to totally different people. In fact, the weekend that I concluded that I needed to totally change my diet and lifestyle, Jeremy was on a Church retreat. At first, I was afraid to tell him of our weekend decision because he had to spend summers with a father who is vegetarian and Jeremy has always returned with horror stories of tofu pizza and beet–carrot juice. But when he came home that weekend he couldn't wait to tell me that he had only eaten salads during the entire retreat. So when I told him of my decision he was all ready for the change.

Now just that tends to put us in a different category than most families. But this is what Jeremy and I call a "God–thing." You see, we firmly believe that knowing that GOD has called us to live and eat healthier is the best motivation to stay with the program. It is much easier to pass a Burger King when you believe you are doing something God has called you to do. Even Jeremy tells his skeptical friends that if God tells you to stop eating meat, then you stop eating meat.

So what do I feed my "Veggie–Boy"?

Well, breakfast is much simpler now—Barleygreen. He drinks his in orange juice most often. But when he is wrestling he mixes it with water and drinks it about 20 minutes before he wrestles.

[I have to interject and say that Dr. Malkmus and I urge Jeremy not to have his Barleygreen in orange juice since the acidity of the OJ neutralizes much of the benefit of the highly alkaline Barleygreen—you get the best results having it in the distilled water, Jeremy…though some would say it doesn't taste as good!—Chet]

For lunch I pack him a bag of one of every fruit we have in the house—oranges, bananas, apples. Sometimes I add a treat of trail mix, mini rice cakes, and/or dried veggies (we get a brand here called "veggibles," which are seasoned with teriyaki, chili or barbecue). The kids teased him at the first when he pulled out trail mix or carrot sticks to nibble on in classes where everyone else was eating cookies, but they got used to it eventually. When he isn't in training or wrestling, I add a cucumber sandwich which includes whole wheat bread, cukes, tomatoes, mushrooms, onions, sprouts, and a spread of hummus or avocado. I also stress the need for water (we don't distill, but we do use/make reverse osmosis water). I make sure he has a LARGE water bottle and that he finishes it before the day is over.

When he first comes home from school he has just ended a two and a half hour wrestling practice and he is *starving*. Then it's time for a smoothie made with orange juice and frozen bananas. If we can afford it, I let him take a second dose of Barleygreen (but using a second jar in a month is sometimes a stretch for our budget). Another snack he likes is hummus (garbanzo bean spread) on whole wheat crackers or matzos. He can also have a second banana or apple at this time. At first he seemed to be hungry all the time, but it appears that the longer we stay with this diet the less hungry both of us are. Also, as a wrestler trying to maintain his weight, he has learned which foods naturally increase his metabolism so he can eat and still lose or maintain his weight. These include oranges (not juiced) and honey (in small amounts). When he has a tournament, I try to fill his bag with plenty of fruit, a honey bottle, rice cakes, and a special treat of a Tiger Milk bar with carob.

For supper we try to stick to Dr. Malkmus's suggestion of a large green salad and then our cooked food. I am fortunate to have a son who loves his veggies so I fill the salad with everything I have in the vegetable bin. For salad dressing we get our favorites from the health food store, always checking for sugar, chemicals and dairy products. But many times he is content to eat his salad without any dressing at all.

For cooked food we will occasionally stray—but being full is often the bigger priority. Jeremy loves baked sweet potatoes so that is usually on the menu at least once a week. But other favorites include veggie chili, baked potatoes covered with vegan chili, homemade soups with any veggies I didn't use in the salad, burritos made with "Just Like Ground," almond cheese mac and cheese, spaghetti, whole wheat pancakes topped with fruit and REAL maple syrup, and Pizza Hut's "The Edge" pizza with all veggies and no cheese. The health food store also has a wonderful variety of vegetarian hot pockets, soups, and no–cheese veggie pizzas.

It's hard to fill up on carrot sticks so we have supplemented with natural peanut butter [*Dr. Malkmus and I would substitute almond butter—Chet*] on whole wheat and sometimes a banana, air–popped popcorn with honey, dried fruit, and an occasional treat of Tofutti or Rice Dream "ice cream." We've also found whole wheat tortillas which are an important staple here in Texas. Those we top with almond cheese, honey, roasted veggies, organic salsa, or nothing at all and warm in the oven. And I make our own granola with oats, coconut, wheat germ, nuts, etc. That can be mixed with dried fruit, carob chips or rolled with natural peanut butter *[or almond butter—Chet]* for a great treat.

For cooked evening meals I have altered all my favorite soup recipes from chicken broth to veggie broth. I still make the best tortilla soup, cabbage soup and various bean soups. And for mashed potatoes I use Rice Dream and just a tad of organic butter (our only animal product in the house, but we use it so seldom a pound lasts two months now). I keep pasta and rice cooked and ready to re–heat and store as many bags of beans as I can fit in the cabinets. I have to admit I still combine rice and beans—guess that's a "Texas" thing.

As I've been writing this I've tried to look over in the kitchen to see what we eat the most of, but I think I've covered it all.

Oh, eating out. Of course, being a teenager my son loves to go out with his friends. The first couple months he would be sure to stop at a store and make a salad from the salad bar so he could eat that while his friends downed hamburgers. He also has the habit now of carrying fruit with him to church so he can eat with his friends if they go out. He has been successful in convincing them to eat at SouperSalad on occasion. We have gradually discovered places that have veggie or black bean burgers on whole wheat buns. One place even lets you get any of their burger combinations with a veggie patty substitute at no extra charge. Subway makes a nice all–veggie sub sandwich, but you have to be careful of the dressing. Most of the grocery stores have salad bars and baked potatoes for a change. Not having fast food to rely on has probably been the biggest challenge since we are an extremely busy family with two drivers and only one car. But we have both gotten to the place where we would rather skip a meal than to cheat. I try to be sure I have fruit with us just in case we can't find anything healthy.

Well, this has gone on quite a while, but I know that when we started this way of life in September I couldn't find enough to read for feeding a teenager. I hope this helps. Just for fun I'm going to add a recipe myself that we love here in Texas. This used to be a once a week soup made with chicken and broth, but this veggie version is actually better.

• • •

Kathleen's Veggie Tortilla Soup

    6 cups vegetable broth
    1 pkg of taco seasoning (from the health food store; no chemical additives, etc.)
    1 cup each of the following dried beans (soaked the night before):
    kidney, black, pinto, red and one can of ranch style NOT drained
    1 can of golden hominy
    1 can stewed tomatoes
    1 can Rotel tomatoes
Cook together for 30 minutes or more and then serve with organic blue corn tortilla chips (from health food store)

No More Kosher Chicken Soup?

(For Women's Eyes Only)
by Kathleen Gabrielle

Let me tell you what I was doing the first time I listened to Dr. Malkmus talk about chickens. Although we are not a Jewish family, my involvement with the Jewish community and Messianic Jews in the area led us to be Kosher. And being a good Kosher cook it wasn't unusual for me to make a weekly stock of chicken broth for soups.

So, having purchased a 10–pound bag of chicken quarters I was doing my weekly boil, de–bone, and freeze. I was also listening to Dr. Malkmus for the first time from his tape on "You don't have to be sick." Just when the aroma of homemade chicken soup had filled my apartment I heard him say that a chicken that used to mature in sixteen weeks now matures in four weeks. I was just about to place a chunk of hot chicken leg piece in my mouth when he mentions that little girls now go into puberty several years early because of all the hormones in chicken. Just to add confirmation to my stubbornness I attempted to make and EAT the chicken soup that night because I "didn't want to waste 10 pounds of chicken," but it tasted horrible.

For the past eight years I have been suffering from menstrual periods that were so heavy I would routinely miss one or two days of work each month. Buying *Always* pads for the month meant filling up a grocery cart. And life was suspended for several days including no karate, biking, standing, walking, working, etc. Two years ago my OB/GYN put me on birth control pills in hopes of controlling my periods, knowing the cost of surgery was not in my budget nor a real desire on his part.

But I was getting so tired of the hassle I would have signed up for an operation in a milli–second. Unfortunately, I was unaware that many birth control pills destroy lysine in the body. That small complication put me on the path to having a flare–up of shingles which lasted several months. I was taking extra doses of lysine, but since I was still on the birth control pills it wasn't helping with the shingles.

That is when I decided to stop taking the birth control pills and try to treat my periods naturally. I began taking evening primrose oil along with several other supplements recommended by ladies at the health food store.

Even though there was a slight improvement, it wasn't enough, and I started asking for a hysterectomy for my 43rd birthday.

That's where I was when first introduced to the Hallelujah Diet and Dr. Malkmus' tapes. It was September 20, 1997, and the results of being chicken–free are worth it all.

In four months I have gone from using 4–5 packages of *Always* a month to one. I have no more cramps. I have no more days of flooding to keep me confined to my bathroom. In fact, my period starts so casually now that I am usually caught by surprise that it has started at all. And I *think* my son would testify that my PMS symptoms have simmered down. I am not taking any supplements. I no longer live on Ibuprofen. I actually have the freedom that you see on stupid Tampax ads.

Some ladies asked why I didn't mention beef. Well, because of pressure concerning fat and cholesterol, we had cut beef out of our diet nearly twelve years ago. But we substituted it with chicken and ground turkey. So for the whole time I was having problems I was ignorantly filling my system with mega–hormones put in today's fowl.

The students I teach all know they can win me over with an apple, but I really get on the girls who devour large frozen dinners full of chicken. "That's gross, Ms. G!" they scream, but I never give up.

I'm not saying that giving up chicken will solve *all* female problems, but I know it did for me. At any rate, it is certainly worth a try if you are anything like I used to be.

The bottom line is that God wants us healthy so we can spend our energy doing the things He has called us to do—whether it is ministry, being a better mom, or telling all our friends how to live longer, healthier lives.

How to cut chicken out of your recipes:

Being an avid soup maker I was saddened to think my famous chicken soup recipes would no longer be enjoyed. But I have discovered that simply substituting vegetable broth for chicken broth and using Bragg Liquid Aminos makes an even better soup with no guilt.

And my favorite chicken fajitas have now been supplanted with roasted veggie fajitas. No, there isn't a true substitute for that traditional Thanksgiving turkey (although we enjoyed lentil loaf with mashed potatoes on top) but knowing that I am feeling so much better the *entire* month motivates me to give up a temporary flesh–satisfier.

What about organic poultry?

Well, I suppose you could try it for families that absolutely insist on having an occasional turkey or chicken. But frankly, I haven't tried this. I figure I've come this far without it so why tempt my taste buds with something I really don't need?

• • •

Tomorrow is the next to the last day of our contract, and I'm going to start pulling the three weeks together at that time. I have some more great letters to share too.

Day Twenty of Our Twenty–One Days to Health the Hallelujah Diet Way

I bet some of you feel like John Glenn getting ready to go back into space again.

Think for a moment about how he must feel—76 years old and about to do what he's probably dreamed of doing every night of his life for decades.

Well, thanks to the Hallelujah Diet and lifestyle, most of us are going to be in the kind of shape when we're 76 that a little ole trip into space will be like a stroll through the park.

Wow, isn't it great?

I love to read stories of men and women in their so–called "golden years" who are actually out there living life to the fullest and having more fun at 70 and 80 than they had at 30 and 40.

Sadly, you don't read those stories very often.

My friends, in the future, as whole generations of us rejuvenate our bodies with the Hallelujah Diet and living by God's natural laws, we're going to not only be reading those stories—they're going to be written about us.

Hallelujah!

I think of the hundreds of thousands of old people in our society who are leading lives of quiet desperation, whose bodies are trembling and shaking from the ravages of the drugs they've taken for years to "control" their various illnesses, whose minds are feeble and unclear—and I want to cry because it *doesn't have to be this way.*

God built into us the capacity to live healthy and happy lives until it was His time for us to go quietly and peacefully in our sleep.

He did not design us to live on "life support systems" that stuck tubes and needles in our bodies.

He did not design us to take five pills in the morning to get going and another five at night to get to sleep.

He did not design us to require yearly check–ups from men and women in white coats, who would then tell us whether or not we were healthy.

Science, modern medicine, and greed designed this model, and look at what it's doing to us, our children, our mothers and fathers, and our grandparents.

Well, it's high time we took responsibility for our own lives and for our own health, and I can't tell you how pumped up I am here on Day Twenty as I write the next to the last contract newsletter and think about the future each of us has thanks to this experience with the Hallelujah Diet.

My friend, I am, for once, literally wordless.

Happily, many others express in their wonderful testimonies of healing and life improvements the same joy Dr. Malkmus and I feel every day.

May I share a few more of these great stories in the rest of today's letter?

• • •

I haven't felt this good since 1995 when I first felt the symptoms of CFIDS and Fibromyalgia coming on. I have a lot more energy, my mind feels clear, and I am closer to God than ever before.

Hey, I was even able to walk one mile on my treadmill, lift light weights and do a few stretching exercises the day before yesterday and I'm ready today to do it again!

I haven't been able to go out late at night because my fatigue felt like a dragon of gloom. But on Wednesday evening I was able to go to a meeting with my husband and we didn't get home until 10:30 p.m. And I STILL felt good! Quite remarkable, to say the least.

Oh, I almost forgot the best part. About four days into the diet I went to a health food store to look for Barleygreen. They did not carry AIM Barleygreen, so I knew I had to keep looking. Two days later I contacted my friend who has lung cancer to tell her about Barleygreen. She said she had just heard about it from an acquaintance and the next thing I know, her friend is on my doorstep with the product in hand. Miracles NEVER cease.

• • •

Chet, after surgery in August, 1996 to remove an ovarian tumor that turned out to be cancerous I was given Dr. Malkmus' book God's Way to Ultimate Health. *Fortunately I read it before submitting to chemotherapy. To make a long story shorter, the doctors thought I was crazy and so did my family and friends when I refused to have any treatment. Instead, I started the Hallelujah diet.*

I went whole hog right off the bat and felt so much better right away that there should have been no question in my mind that this was the right thing to be doing. But everyone I tried to explain this to questioned my sanity. I started to feel that I wasn't doing enough to bolster my immune system. Every time I got scared and was about to do chemo, I'd read Dr. Malkmus' book again! I'd be sure again until I heard one more horror story.

I'm sure there are people out there who can relate to what I've been going through. What I wouldn't have given to have had this service that you are providing now.

There was a person who gave a testimonial in the book who lived in my state. I was able to locate her and get some help. My first question to her was "Are these people online? I have so many questions that I wish I could e–mail." Imagine my excitement when I got the news that Hallelujah Acres was online at www.hacres.com

I lost 55 lbs., jog two to three miles almost every day, never get sick and STILL friends will ask, with that very concerned look, how I'm feeling. I must admit that I still get concerned on occasion as to whether or not I am cancer free. I have to have a great deal of faith and commitment. I praise God and thank everyone there for their commitment to getting the truth out about God's way to ultimate health. There is so much resistance. I thought my life itself would be proof enough, but most people really don't want to make any sacrifices. I tell people that the only thing I've sacrificed is the discomfort associated with poor health! Hallelujah!! I also want people to know that if

I'd read Dr. Malkmus' book before I had surgery, I would have tried the diet and not even had surgery!

• • •

I was diagnosed the first week of December '97 with colon cancer... Our Pastor's wife was talking to some acquaintances of hers (actually Hallelujah Acres Health Ministers) about the Hallelujah Diet because her dad is sick. She told me about the Hallelujah Diet that Sunday morning and we met your Health Ministers after the service.

So the first week in December we started the complete Hallelujah Diet. That week was terrible. All we seemed to do was wash, juice, clean up, cut veggies, eat, drink the juice and Barleygreen, go to bed, then get up and repeat the process. I had many pity parties that week, trying to come to terms with my diagnosis and my future. I had decided not to have surgery (Lord, am I doing the right thing?) and all the other stuff the doctors wanted to do to me.

Well, the Lord showered us with His blessings. We were given a Champion juicer and a large water distiller. Another friend introduced us to a local carrot farmer where we get 50 lbs. of carrots for a $1.00. I decided I'd trust God to use this new way of eating to heal me of cancer.

I've lost 12 lbs. so far, and continue feeling good. Everyone says I'm "perky." I feel perky. Some old clothes I have, now fit me again!

Most importantly, prior to our starting the HDiet, I would have at least four or five migraines a month—some of them severe enough to put me to bed, when I wasn't throwing up, for up to two to three days. (Medication was costing about $100 a month.) My headaches were caused by climatic changes, stress, and combinations of certain foods (although I was managing the food triggers quite well). I had received prayer many, many, many times, but God chose not to heal the migraines completely.

But guess what, folks? I have not had a headache since I've been on the Hallelujah Diet. Praise the Lord! Actually, that's not quite true. I had a pressure headache one night. It was 8:00 p.m and we hadn't eaten. So I went to get dinner (veggies of course) and took my carrot juice and BG. Suddenly, I realized that within five minutes my headache was gone. Wow! Talk about my cells yelling WHOOPEE!

So we are thanking God for using His diet to get rid of my migraines. I'm convinced that, if I went back on the Standard American Diet, they would recur. BUT, why would I do that?

One of our friends suggested that because our HD diet is "so extreme," that maybe "when we get better" we could go back to eating "normally." We asked her: "Why would we go back to eating something that made us sick in the first place?" But, she couldn't see it. We relate to the Day 17 Newsletter [see page 74], Chet.

It is beyond us how people who are sick can totally reject the Hallelujah Lifestyle. We are convinced because of our experience that some people are used to being sick and are afraid to be well. Sickness is the only thing they know and so many things would change if they were well. And also how could something so simple "cure" diseases that the medical establishment cannot. But, as you say, we cannot jam it down people's throats. (If we did, though, they would be healthier).

• • •

Today's recipe from Rhonda Malkmus:

• • •

Seasoned Basmati Rice

This is one of our favorites on a cold winter evening after we have had our Barleygreen and salad. This is the only kind of rice we use and the aroma of this rice cooking will tantalize your taste buds.

1 cup brown Basmati rice, rinsed and set aside
1/2 cup of celery, chopped
1/4 cup onion chopped
1/4 cup red and/or green pepper
3 cups distilled water

Sauté the celery, onion and peppers in water, vegetable soup stock or olive oil, until onion is translucent. Add rice and sauté a few minutes (do not let it burn). Then add three cups of distilled water and bring quickly to a boil. Cover, reduce heat and simmer for 30 minutes. Turn burner off and allow to sit covered an additional 15 to 30 minutes. Do not lift lid. Stir, season with Bragg Liquid Aminos and herbs to taste. Serve alone or use as a base on which to place stir–fried or steamed vegetables.

• • •

Today's joke comes courtesy of my friend Ronn:

A man was very upset when his dog just rolled over and stopped breathing. He rushed him to the vet, who examined the dog briefly and announced, "I'm sorry, but your dog is dead."

"Isn't there anything more you can do?" the guy asked.

The vet said there was something else he could try, and he laid the dog on a table. He brought in a box, placed it next to the dog, took off the lid, and a cat jumped out. The cat walked up to the dog, looked at it, walked all around it, sniffed it a couple of times, then got back in the box.

"Well, that's it, your dog is dead," said the vet. "That will be $350.00"

The man was shocked! "$350.00 for WHAT?" he demanded.

"Well," the vet replied, "$50 for the office visit, and $300 for the cat scan."

• • •

Tomorrow we'll pull it all together! See you then for the last day of our 21–Days to Health the Hallelujah Diet Way.

Final Day of Our Twenty–One Days to Health the Hallelujah Diet Way

Well, my friend, the day we've been looking forward to has finally arrived. Day Twenty–One, the end of the contract.

If you've been faithful to the program and have worked it with all its components—daily juicing, daily Barleygreen, daily raw fruits and veggies, daily exercise, and so on—chances are you feel a whole lot better than when you started.

You've also lost at least five pounds and probably a lot more than that.

You probably have an energy level that's significantly better than three short weeks ago.

You may well be sleeping sounder and waking up earlier.

You're probably thinking more clearly and feeling more emotionally grounded and calm.

Your I.Q. has gone up to 173.

Just kidding on that one.

I could spend this entire letter listing benefits, but I'll stop with the main ones which I trust most of you have experienced, at least in one degree or another.

Please remember, however, that degree is important here.

Not all people heal at the same rate, and three weeks is a very short time to overcome the toxic problems that have taken you a lifetime to develop.

This is one of the reasons Dr. Malkmus encourages folks to take the Hallelujah Diet challenge for a full 90–days.

You see, most bodies don't even come close to detoxing in three quick weeks.

But in three weeks most people will see enough positive changes to encourage them to continue. And that's what Dr. Malkmus and I strongly encourage you to do: extend your contract and go for the 90–day challenge on your own.

You've made a great start—why stop now?

Please, don't celebrate your contract victory tonight by going out for a steak with onion rings and a slice of cheese cake.

Why not?

Two reasons.

First, that stuff's not fuel for the body.

If you still think meat is good for you, please log on to the Internet and point your browser to *http://hacres.com/html/cannibal.html* to see what that juicy steak really contains.

Second, eating that stuff right after twenty–one days of feeding your body the right way is going to make you feel awful.

Oh, it may (and I say may because it also may not) taste good at first, but trust me when I tell you it's gonna make you feel bad an hour or so after you eat it, and it's going to make you feel even worse the next day.

Most people I know on the Hallelujah Diet will get bad headaches or stomach aches from eating flesh after they've been off it for a few weeks—and that's because of all the hormones and antibiotics and dyes and Lord knows what else is in the highly processed meat produced by the flesh merchants.

My friend, I didn't tell you this when we started, but there's no going back once you've been on God's diet for a few weeks. Oh sure, you can slowly and gradually slip back into Standard American Diet SADness, but it'll never be quite the same.

Because every time you're constipated, every time you get a headache, every time your belly hurts, every time you're crabby and snapping at your kids, every time you get depressed—you're going to know in your heart that you've *caused* your own problem by eating incorrectly.

Knowledge is wonderful, but it cuts two ways, and now that you have the knowledge of "How not to be sick," it's your responsibility to your body/temple to use that knowledge for your own good.

It goes even further than that.

You also have the responsibility to share this knowledge with friends, loved ones, and even acquaintances and strangers.

The world's not going to rush to make this knowledge available because it would upset too many major industries that make their money off human misery.

So we're not going to hear about this on the nightly news—the news will keep us stupefied with "breaking stories" about the sex lives of politicians and other non–stories the media moguls want to dumb us down with.

But, hey, they can't stop us from sharing the truth among ourselves, can they?

And Dr. Malkmus and I know that we as individuals, one person at a time, can spread the knowledge and "how to do it" specifics of the Hallelujah Diet. With this knowledge, each of us can help our brothers and sisters free themselves of chronic medical problems that are keeping them in pain and in debt, in many cases.

How do you share this knowledge?

It's easy.

Talk to folks who are curious about what you've just done. When they see you looking better, when they see you energetic and happy, when they see you laughing all the time, that's when people will want to know what you've done to bring about all these positive changes.

Then you can tell them you've discovered this new lifestyle that rejuvenates the body and the spirit.

If their eyes start to glaze over, back off.

But if they want to know more, give them the details, and if they want to test our program, loan them a copy of this book so they can go on twenty–one days to health for themselves.

Also share with them a copy of our *Back to the Garden* magazine or point them to our web site at *http://www.hacres.com* where they can find all the information they need on how and why they should live by the Hallelujah Diet.

Some folks won't make it, of course, due to lack of discipline or busy lives or unsupportive family or failure to work the program the way it's taught or whatever, but many will make it, and these folks can then go out and share the good news with others as well.

My friend, we are a groundswell, a snowball rolling down a huge mountain, an avalanche of good news waiting to happen.

If each of us does a small part, we can begin to heal a sick and suffering world.

So, please, share what you've learned with anyone who will listen.

If you have really been touched by the diet during the past twenty–one days and if you think you might want to do more than casually share the information with others, you may want to become one of our health ministers. If you feel called to learn everything you can about the Hallelujah Diet and lifestyle, you may want to attend one of Dr. Malkmus' two and a half day training sessions.

For details on our health ministry program and how to apply for our information packet, set your browser to: *http://hacres.com/html/ministry.html* or else write us at the address on page 102 of this book and request our health ministry packet.

Whatever you do in terms of sharing the "You don't have to be sick" message, we thank you in advance for doing it.

Finally, a few words on the topic of additional support. Although due to the volume of e–mail we can't promise to personally answer every letter we receive at Hallelujah Acres, we do publish a weekly *Hallelujah Health Tip* on the Internet. To get a free subscription to this informative and highly entertaining publication, just send an e–mail to *subscribe@hacres.com* and we'll sign you right up.

We're also looking at some other support options, and I'll update you on these possibilities in the *Hallelujah Health Tip* as time goes by.

And remember, I check my e–mail seven days a week, and you can always write to *chet@hacres.com* if you need a little personal encouragement. I don't promise a long, detailed reply, but I will have at least a few words for you within 24–hours after receiving your letter.

Okay, how about one last fabulous testimony, one that nicely summarizes the great results that come to so many when they follow the Hallelujah Diet:

• • •

Dear Chet,

I have to thank you from the bottom of my heart for turning me on to this new way of life. I was extremely skeptical at first, but decided I'd give it a try. I was extremely depressed, always tired, no energy, and crabby all the time. My husband, kids and friends have been very impressed to see me becoming my old self again! I am happy all the time, I don't get angry or upset easily like before, I have a ton of energy, and have now been told I'm "a lot of fun again." My witty sense of humor has come back, my love and zest for life is back, and for the first time in about nine years, I have a very positive outlook on life and the world around me! You've truly given me back my life.... It was great that it was just starting out as a 21–day contract because I don't believe I would have tried it if it had been longer. Of course, I will not go back to my SAD eating ways, but three weeks ago, I just thought I'd eat well for three weeks and then that'd be that. I will be trying to show people how they can improve their lives. My husband is already considering it now and when I started this three weeks ago, he thought I was crazy. But, he now sees how great of a difference it has made in me. I'm gradually putting my children onto this way of eating as well, a bit at a time. I wish that everyone in this world would be willing to put their skepticism aside for just three weeks and try this new way of life. We could wipe out illness, and, if people's personalities improved as much as mine, we'd truly all be living in a much better world.

• • •

Finally, I have to tell you that I've had more fun the past three weeks while writing these daily tips than I think I've had at any other time in my life. It's been a remarkable period, and I hope you share my joy in the success we have shared.

I thank you for participating in Twenty—One Days to Health the Hallelujah Diet Way. God bless you.

P.S. Below I list just some of the ailments that men and women reported as either improved or totally healed during our Twenty—One Day online contract challenge in January of 1998. Just for fun, circle the ones that fit for you.

Increased energy	Lost lots of weight	No more dry scalp
Enhanced mental clarity	Greater stamina	Less irritable
Fatigue reduced	Skin improved	More poise
Back pain gone	Constipation gone	Sinus infections gone
Shrinking hemorrhoids	Shrinking prostate	Less body odor
Improved strength	Less joint pain	No more migraines
Eczema almost gone	Better vision	Speedier healing
Arthritis improved	Itching gone	No more sugar cravings
Heart palpitations gone	Insomnia gone	Menstrual cramps gone
Congestion improved	Sluggishness gone	Eating a lot less
Need less sleep	Chest pain gone	Gastroparesis improved
Complexion clearer	Blood pressure better	Less stomach pain
No more indigestion	Low energy gone	Skin cancer smaller
Asthma gone	Dry skin gone	No more heartburn
Bowel problems gone	Mood swings gone	Improved coordination
Brighter eyes	Spider veins fading	Gums healed—teeth tighter
Hot flashes gone	Less bloating	Desire for alcohol gone

The Hallelujah Diet
by Rev. George H. Malkmus

People often ask me, "What do you eat?" Here is my answer:

Breakfast
One tablespoon of BARLEYGREEN* powder either dry and let it dissolve in my mouth or in a couple ounces of distilled water at room temperature. That is usually all I have until noon. If I do get hungry, then I may eat a piece of fresh juicy fruit later in the morning. Cooked food is an absolute no–no as my body is in a cleansing mode until about noon each day. (It is vitally important to me that the BARLEYGREEN powder I use comes from AMERICAN IMAGE MAR-KETING and that it contains kelp. There are other companies that have tried to imitate this product, but they are not processed the same way. I have tried other products, but they do not give the same results. Nor do the BARLEYGREEN caplets if swallowed. The caplets can be dissolved in the mouth like a lozenge, however. I enjoy them in this form, especially while travelling.)

Lunch
One tablespoon of BARLEYGREEN* powder, as at breakfast. Sometimes I stir my BARLEYGREEN into 8 ounces of freshly extracted carrot juice**, which I find especially delicious and extremely nutritious. At least a half hour after the BARLEYGREEN, I prefer an all–raw fruit lunch. A banana, apple, dates, etc. Organic is always best when available. (Sometimes I have a vegetable salad for lunch instead of the fruit.) It is important that this be an all raw meal!

Supper
One tablespoon of BARLEYGREEN* powder either dry or in a couple ounces of distilled water or in carrot juice. Carrot juice must be freshly extracted, never powdered, canned, bottled, or frozen. Then, at least 30 minutes after the BARLEYGREEN, I eat a large green vegetable salad of leaf lettuce (never head lettuce), broccoli, cauliflower, celery, carrots, etc. This is usually followed by some cooked food (baked potato, baked sweet potato, brown rice, steamed vegetables, whole–grain pasta, whole–grain bread, etc.) Later in the evening I often have a glass of organic apple juice or a piece of juicy fruit. (My diet consists of approximately 85 percent raw food, and 15 percent cooked food.)

To be sure I get the essential fatty acids needed by my body, I also have one tablespoon of a cold–pressed, organic flax seed oil. I either have this on my evening salad or straight out of the bottle.

Exercise is also an essential part of my program. I do at least one hour of vigorous exercise daily. Additionally, I try to get some sunshine on as much of my body as possible every day.

*The reason I supplement my diet with BARLEYGREEN is that our food today is being grown for the most part in very deficient soils that often lack all the nutrients my body needs for building new, strong, healthy, vital, vibrant cells. BARLEYGREEN is grown organically and contains the widest spectrum of nutrients available today from a single source that I am aware of. It is also loaded with enzymes. I consider it the single, most important food I put into my body each day and always consume at least three tablespoons of it a day. Another AIM product we find very beneficial is Herbal Fiberblend, for added fiber, preventative maintenance of the colon and insurance against parasitic infestations. I take one tablespoon a day and Rhonda takes two tablespoons.

**The second–most important thing I put into my body each day is freshly extracted carrot juice made from large California juicing carrots. I try to drink at least 16 to 24 ounces each day. When I had my colon cancer in 1976, I consumed 32 to 64 ounces of carrot juice each day. If I had a serious physical problem today I would consume up to eight 8–ounce glasses of carrot juice each day in addition to my three to four tablespoons of Barleygreen. I would have four 8–ounce servings of juice between my breakfast Barleygreen and lunch and four more 8–ounce servings between lunch and supper. I would have these servings of juice at one hour intervals. The reason Barleygreen and carrot juice is so important to me is:

1. Cooked food has practically no nutritional value.
2. A large percentage of the nutrients in raw food are lost in the digestion process, with only 1 to 35% of nutrients reaching cell level, depending on the health of the digestive system.
3. When vegetable juices or Barleygreen is consumed, up to 92% of the nutrients reach cell level. This is because the pulp has been removed and thus no digestion is necessary. Raw vegetable juices are the fastest way to nourish the cells and rebuild the body.
4. If I had cancer I would not have fruit (Nathan Pritikin, Dr. Stanley Bass, and the macrobiotics believe that fruit sugar helps to spread cancer). If I had candida, I would not have fruit or carrot juice (because of the high glycemic index). If I had diabetes, I would monitor my blood sugar very carefully while transitioning to the Hallelujah Acres program.
5. We encourage individuals with chronic health challenges who want to try the Hallelujah Diet to work with a *nutritionally–minded physician* who has knowledge of our program. If your doctor doesn't know about our program, give him a copy of *Back to the Garden* and encourage him/her to read it and discuss it with you. If your doctor then tells you the diet is dangerous, ask why so many people report in our magazine of being healed of so many different ailments with our program? If your doctor can't provide a satisfactory answer, you may want to seek out a physician who has a better understanding of the nutrition/disease connection.

Hallelujah Acres Health Resources

BARLEYGREEN is an organically grown, live food from the juice of young barley leaves. The juice is spray–dried in a vacuum at room temperature in two seconds, resulting in a bright green powder very rich in vitamins, minerals, live enzymes, chlorophyll and protein. Barleygreen is the most nutritionally–dense food ever found, providing one of the widest spectrums of naturally–occurring nutrients available. There are other barley products on the market, but this is the only one we have found that gives truly miraculous results. Comes in a 7–ounce jar, containing 66 teaspoons. Barleygreen is the only nutritional supplement Rhonda and I take. We cannot recommend it highly enough!!! ($33.95 for 7–oz. jar)

BARLEYGREEN in New Family–Size Jar AIM is now offering a 10.5–ounce plastic jar of Barleygreen. ($49.95 for 10.5 oz)

HERBAL FIBERBLEND is the result of over twenty years of study and personal experiences of many users. This careful study and consideration has combined selected herbs and fiber for maximum contribution to the daily diet. Contains seventeen different herbs in a psyllium base. Each herb is placed in the blend for a specific purpose (e.g. Shavegrass and Black Walnut hulls kill eggs of parasites and expels parasites; Pumpkin Seed is good for prostate problems; Licorice Root is a tonic for the intestinal tract, stimulating enzymes and peristaltic action; Slippery Elm coats the digestive tract and aids in healing inflammation, etc.) Raspberry flavor (#401) comes in a 16–oz. size & lemon flavor (#413) comes in a 12–oz. size. Indicate the flavor you want. Rhonda and I use this product every day and highly recommend it! ($32.95)

WHY CHRISTIANS GET SICK by Dr. George Malkmus is very helpful in introducing Christians to a natural diet and lifestyle. Letters are received daily from all over the world from people helped by this book, which is now in its 20th printing. Why Christians Get Sick is written on a solid Biblical foundation with over 150 Bible verses. This was Dr. Malkmus' first book. (Paperback, $8.95)

GOD'S WAY TO ULTIMATE HEALTH by Dr. George Malkmus with Michael Dye has everything you need to know about how to return to God's original plan for nourishing the human body. Read what the Bible says about diet and how this Biblical wisdom is supported by modern science and hundreds of real–life testimonials. Also an entire section of recipes and tips by Rhonda Malkmus on how to set up your own natural foods kitchen. God's Way to Ultimate Health contains 282 pages of vital information that has changed the way thousands of people think about what they put into their bodies. Many people say this book has saved their lives. (Perfect bound paperback, $18.95)

RECIPES FOR LIFE…FROM GOD'S GARDEN by Rhonda Malkmus is the perfect companion piece to God's Way to Ultimate Health because it begins where the theory and rationale for the diet leaves off. With more than 400 nutritious and delicious recipes, our prayer is that this huge 8 1/2 by 11–inch spiral bound book will eventually be treasured in every kitchen in the land. Healthy food tastes wonderful, and this book proves it. Has important chapters on how to feed children and young adults, along with menus and even a section on feeding babies. Detailed index lists recipes not only by chapter but also alphabetically. (Spiral bound, $24.95)

THE CHAMPION JUICER—This is a masticating juicer, which breaks up the cells and fibers of food, forcing its nutritional value into the juice. We do not recommend any juicer with a spinning basket because it only shreds the food, leaving much of the nutrients in the pulp. The Champion is extremely well–made, is easy to clean, runs smoothly and quietly and has a 1–year limited warranty on motor and 5 years on juicing parts. In addition to juicing fruits and vegetables, you can make banana ice cream, baby food, nut butters and more. 25 lbs., 17" l., 8" w, 13" h. (Regularly $289.00, our price $269.00, including shipping.)

GREEN POWER JUICE EXTRACTOR—This juicer offers several unique features that give it an advantage over other juicers. The Green Power has a twin–gear, low–RPM motor that produces less heat, which minimizes loss of nutrition. The slow–moving triturating twin gears crush the fruits and vegetables, rather than cutting them. The Green Power can also make wheatgrass juice, baby foods, nut butters, pastas, rice cakes, frozen desserts, bean curd and more. This machine expels a drier pulp, an indication that more juice and more nutrients are being extracted. 32 lbs., 20" l., 8" w., 13" h. Rhonda and Dr. Malkmus use this juicer. (Reg. $650.00—Our price: $595.00, including shipping)

HOW TO ELIMINATE SICKNESS VIDEO '97—This professionally–produced video was shot on–site in Eidson, Tennessee, the former home of Hallelujah Acres. The 2 1/2–hour seminar contains much updated information not available in our earlier videotapes, including Bible Scripture and educational text super–imposed over breathtaking views of the rural East Tennessee country-side. This is an updated version of the seminar Dr. Malkmus has delivered across the United States and Canada. It covers the basics of why we get sick and how to nourish our bodies to restore our health. It will change your thinking forever as to what is nutrition and what is not. You must see this remarkable video. ($24.95)

HOW TO ELIMINATE SICKNESS AUDIO '97—This two–cassette audio was taken from the soundtrack of the above 1997 How to Eliminate Sickness Video. This is a dynamic presentation of the health message from a Biblical perspective. This recording has much new information not available in previous recordings. (Two tapes in jacket, $12.95)

REBOUNDER—This high–quality mini–trampoline can offer one of the best indoor low–impact aerobic workouts ever devised. It's a great foul–weather alternative to walking or jogging. Includes a 40–inch diameter heavy–duty metal frame, six spring–loaded legs (removable for easy storage) and it folds in half to fit into its own carrying bag. Please specify hard or soft bounce. The hard bounce, which contains more tension in the springs and membrane, is recommended for people who weigh over 300 lbs. but is not guaranteed by the manufacturer, while the soft bounce is recommended for people less than 300 lbs. and is guaranteed for three years. Used every day by Rhonda and Dr. Malkmus. ($209.00)

TESTIMONIAL VIDEO—Filmed in 1997 at the Tulsa Bible Prophecy Conference, this moving video features five–minute testimonies of 13 men and women who healed themselves of a remarkable variety of illnesses by going on the Hallelujah Diet. This video contains testimonies by a medical doctor, nurses, preachers, and folks from many walks of life. If you know someone who resists the "You don't have to be sick" message, this tape of testimonials will open their hearts to the truth of the power of the Hallelujah Diet. ($14.95)

TWENTY–ONE DAYS TO HEALTH THE HALLELUJAH DIET WAY—In this 104–page book Hallelujah Acres Online editor Chet Day takes you by the hand and shows you how to lose weight and dramatically improve your overall quality of life in three short weeks. Containing daily motivational letters written in Chet's amusing and informative syle, this popular guide shows you how to make the Hallelujah Diet work in your life. Priced so you can buy one for yourself and several for suffering friends and relatives. ($4.95–see order form on next page for quantity discounts)

Hallelujah Acres
PO Box 2388
Shelby NC 28151

Call us at 1–704–481–1700
from 8–5 Monday–Friday and 10–2 (EST) on Saturdays to order.

Or order from our web site at:
http://www.hacres.com

Or use the order form on the next page.

Quantity Discounts—*Twenty-One Days to Health the Hallelujah Diet Way*

Number of Copies	Price	Number of Copies	Price
1–3 books	$4.95 each	4–10 books	$3.96 each
11–49 books	$3.47 each	50–over	$2.97 each

Customer Order Form
Return Policy (Juicers, Distillers, etc.)

If you return an item in new condition with the original warranty intact, we charge a 10% restocking fee. If you return an item in new condition, but without the warranty, we charge a 15% restocking fee. If you return an item in used condition with the original warranty intact, we charge a 15% restocking fee. If you return an item in used condition without the warranty, we charge a 20% restocking fee. Call Peter Malkmus for prior approval before returning any item. Customer pays for all return shipping. Credit will be given after the product is returned and inspected. No refunds after thirty (30) days.

Name: _____

Address: _____

City: _____ State: _____ Zip: _____

Phone: ( ) _____

Please provide a physical address–not a P.O. Box–for UPS delivery.

☐ Please check if you are not on our mailing list, and would like a free subscription to *Back to the Garden.*

Qty.	Item #	Item Name	Price Each	Total

☐ Check ☐ Money Order ☐ Visa ☐ MC
☐ Discover ☐ American Express

Card Number: _____

Signature: _____

Card Exp. Date _____

Sub-total	
6% Sales Tax (NC residents only)	
Shipping	
Total	

Shipping Charges

$5 for all orders under $50. Add 10% for orders over $50. Call for foreign rates outside of the Continental U.S. North Carolina residents, please add 6% sales tax to entire order.

How to Reach Us

Credit Card Orders Call: (704) 481-1700
Mail Orders to:
Hallelujah Acres
P.O. Box 2388
Shelby, NC 28151
Fax: (704) 481-0345 • **Website:** www.hacres.com